Anal and Rectal Diseases

Eli D. Ehrenpreis · Shmuel Avital · Marc Singer
Editors

Anal and Rectal Diseases

A Concise Manual

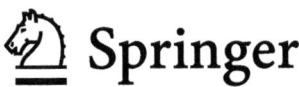 Springer

Editors
Eli D. Ehrenpreis, MD
Chief of Gastroenterology and Endoscopy
Highland Park Hospital
Medical Director, Center for the Study of
Complex Diseases
NorthShore University Health System
Clinical Associate Professor of Medicine
University of Chicago Medical Center
Highland Park, IL, USA

Shmuel Avital, MD
Chief of Surgery
Department of Surgery B
Meir Medical Center
Kfar-Saba, Israel

Marc Singer, MD
NorthShore University Health System
Department of Surgery
Division of Colon and Rectal Surgery
Evanston, IL, USA

ISBN 978-1-4614-1101-7   e-ISBN 978-1-4614-1102-4
DOI 10.1007/978-1-4614-1102-4
Springer New York Dordrecht Heidelberg London

Library of Congress Control Number: 2011939744

Springer is part of Springer Science+Business Media (www.springer.com)

I would like to express my gratitude to my wife Ana for her encouragement, to my children Benjamin, Jamie, and Joseph for their understanding, and to my parents, Bella and Seymour for bringing academics and scholarship to my world.

Eli D. Ehrenpreis, MD

I would like thank my wife, Michal, for her ongoing support since I was a medical student and her understanding of the time commitments involved in academia beyond the obvious time needed for clinical practice.
Shmuel Avital, MD

Preface

Anorectal pathology is common in the general population. Understanding the pathophysiology, diagnosis, and treatment of diseases of the anus and rectum is often quite a challenge for physicians and other healthcare providers. There are many barriers to achievement of high quality care for these conditions. Patients may be embarrassed to admit to anorectal symptoms. Specific education about diseases of the anus and rectum may be limited among primary treating physicians depending on the institution where training takes place. Of most importance from the author's standpoint, a short book that connects together anorectal anatomy and pathophysiology with medical and surgical treatment of anorectal disease is needed by many in the medical field.

In creating *Anal and Rectal Diseases: A Concise Manual*, my surgical coeditors and I have worked diligently to fulfill the aforementioned unmet need. The style of the book was developed to communicate the most important information on each topic in brief, therefore making the book useful for reference and review. Studying a specific chapter will give the reader an accurate overall picture of each subject. We have also included many figures to aid the reader in their understanding of the presented material. By adding detailed information about surgeries performed for these conditions, it is our hope that practitioners who are not surgeons will develop a deeper understanding of these procedures, their indications, their benefits to the patient as well as their potential complications.

Throughout the book, we have included "clinical pearls," generally summarizing important aspects of the preceding short chapter. These small pieces of insight are selected by choice of the individual section authors. They may represent the author's opinion based on experience rather than pure evidence from technical literature about the topic. We believe that despite tremendous advances in the scientific application of medical knowledge, clinical experience, reflected in the practitioner's art, remains a vital dynamic in the complete care of a patient.

Highland Park, IL
Kfar-Saba, Israel
Evanston, IL

Eli D. Ehrenpreis, MD
Shmuel Avital, MD
Marc Singer, MD

Introduction

Anorectal disorders are among the most common problems encountered in primary care practice. These maladies include a wide array of benign and malignant conditions effecting patients of all ages spanning the pediatric to the geriatric groups. Patients frequently present to their primary care provider with such diverse disorders such as fistula and abscess, fissure and stenosis, anal and rectal carcinoma, condylomata acuminata and sexually transmitted diseases, and hemorrhoids. In addition, symptoms ranging from pruritis ani to painless rectal bleeding are cause for analysis by the primary care provider. Due to the prevalence of these problems the primary care provider and trainee require access to a comprehensive, clear, and concise volume to help them with the evaluation and management of these issues. There are a plethora of volumes available to assist the practitioner with the management of anorectal disorders. However, very few of these books are written from the point of view of a gastroenterologist. As surgeons we occasionally, or perhaps routinely, become myopically focused upon a myriad of surgical terminology, descriptions of methodology, and illustrations of techniques.

Therefore, it was very refreshing for me to read some of the chapters in Dr. Ehrenpreis and his coeditors' new book which offer an alternative gastroenterologic perspective on anorectal disorders. The descriptive methods as well as the diagnostic and therapeutic modalities described will be very clinically relevant for the practicing internist, family practitioner, and gastroenterologist as well as the trainees in those areas. I am absolutely confident that this book will be a welcome additional to the clinical library of many primary care practitioners and trainees and as such I highly commend it to gastroenterologists, family practitioners, internists, and interns, residents, and fellows in those specialties who evaluate and manage patients with diseases of the anus and rectum. Given the frequency of such disorders, I can safely recommend this book to all of these practitioners and their respective trainees. I congratulate Dr. Ehrenpreis, Dr. Singer, and Dr. Avital for having gathered this information and arranged and presented it in such an easy to follow manner. I am also honored that they have asked me to write this introduction.

Weston, FL   Steven D. Wexner, MD

Contents

Contributors

Shmuel Avital, MD Chief of Surgery, Department of Surgery B, Meir Medical Center, Kfar-Saba, Israel

Eli D. Ehrenpreis, MD Chief of Gastroenterology and Endoscopy, Highland Park Hospital, NorthShore University Health System, Highland Park, IL 60035, USA

Clinical Associate Professor of Medicine, University of Chicago Medical Center, Highland Park, IL, USA

Ron Greenberg, MD Surgical Division, Tel Aviv Sourasky Medical Center, 10 Weizman Street, Tel Aviv, Israel

Yehuda Kariv, MD Tel Aviv Sourasky Medical Center, Colo-rectal Surgery Unit, Division of Surgery, 10 Weizman Street, Tel Aviv, Israel

Marc Singer, MD Department of Surgery, Division of Colon and Rectal Surgery, NorthShore University Health System, Evanston, IL, USA

Part I
Medical

Chapter 1
General Information

Eli D. Ehrenpreis

Anal and Rectal Anatomy

Anal Canal

The anal canal is the terminal portion of the gastrointestinal tract. It is the short tubular segment, distal to the rectum, which is lined internally by squamous and transitional epithelium. The anal canal begins where the distal rectum penetrates the muscular floor of the pelvic cavity. It is surrounded by the anal sphincter muscle.

Rectum

The rectum is the distal portion of the large intestine. It is defined as the region lying between the sigmoid colon and the anal canal, and is approximately 12–15 cm in length. The lower third of the rectum is distal to the peritoneal reflection. Unlike in the rest of the colon, longitudinal muscle fibers in the rectum do not form discrete lengthwise bands (teniae) but, instead, surround the entire rectum (see Fig. 1.1). The dentate line marks the distal portion of the rectum and separates it from the anal canal (see Fig. 1.2). It also separates two types of epithelia, the simple columnar epithelium of the rectum and the stratified epithelium of the anal canal (anoderm). The dentate line has multiple folds – the columns of Morgagni. The anal crypts and glands are located at

E.D. Ehrenpreis, MD (✉)
Chief of Gastroenterology and Endoscopy, Highland Park Hospital,
NorthShore University Health System, Highland Park, IL 60035, USA

Clinical Associate Professor of Medicine, University of Chicago Medical Center,
Highland Park, IL 60035, USA
e-mail: ehrenpreis@gipharm.net

E.D. Ehrenpreis et al. (eds.), *Anal and Rectal Diseases: A Concise Manual*,
DOI 10.1007/978-1-4614-1102-4_1, © Springer Science+Business Media, LLC 2012

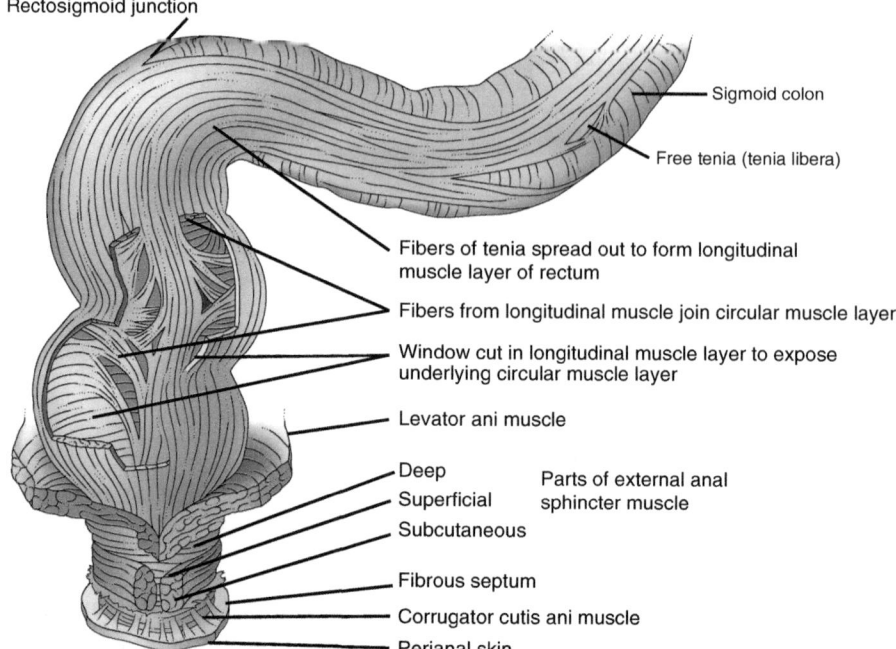

Fig. 1.1 Rectal muscle anatomy

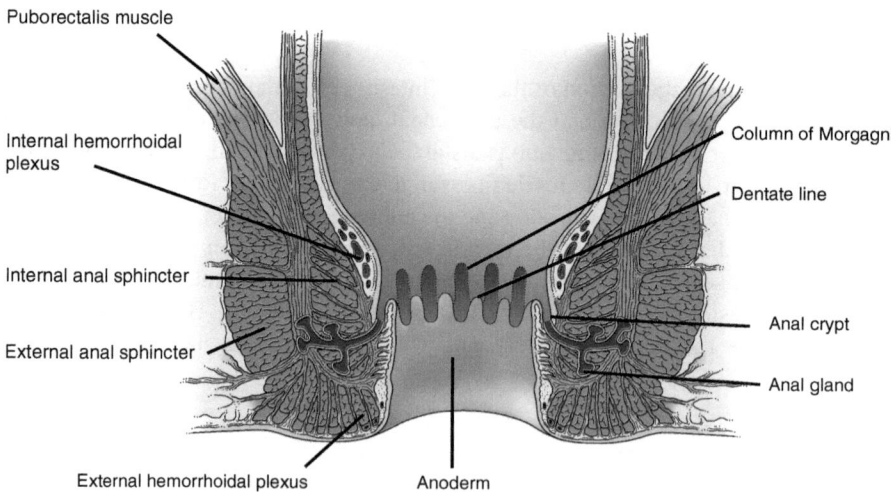

Fig. 1.2 Anatomy of the anal region

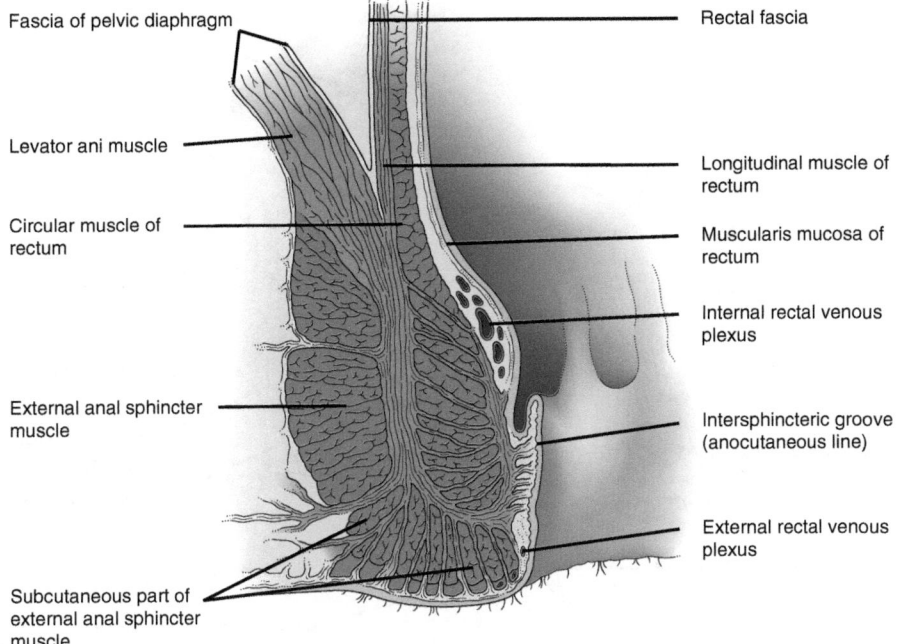

Fascia of pelvic diaphragm

Rectal fascia

Levator ani muscle

Longitudinal muscle of
rectum

Circular muscle of
rectum

Muscularis mucosa of
rectum

Internal rectal venous
plexus

External anal sphincter
muscle

Intersphincteric groove
(anocutaneous line)

External rectal venous
plexus

Subcutaneous part of
external anal sphincter
muscle

Fig. 1.3   Anal muscle anatomy

the base of the columns of Morgagni. These glands may be the site of perianal abscess
and fistula formation. The rectum has three folds, called the valves of Houston.

Musculature

Internal Anal Sphincter

The internal anal sphincter is a thick ring of fibers from the circular smooth muscle
from the colon at the proximal portion of the anal canal (see Figs. 1.2, 1.3).

External Anal Sphincter

The external anal sphincter surrounds the anal canal at the pelvic diaphragm, distal
to the anal orifice (see Fig. 1.3). The external anal sphincter is a ring of skeletal
muscle, which extends superiorly to the puborectalis, an important constituent of
the levator ani, the main muscle of the pelvic floor. Posteriorly, the external anal
sphincter has attachments to the coccyx and, anteriorly, to the perineal body. The
puborectalis muscle attaches anteriorly to the pubic bone and envelops the lower

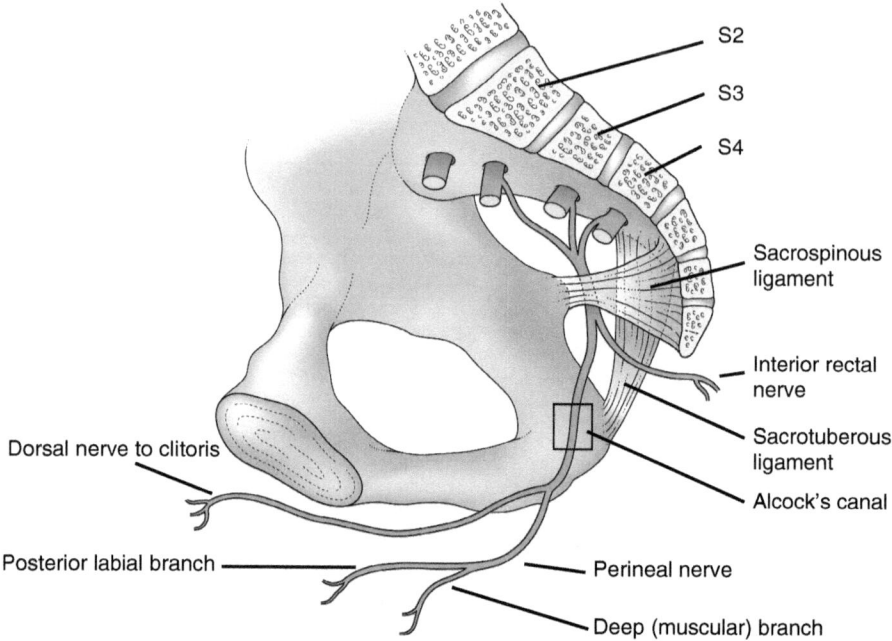

Fig. 1.4 The branches of the pudendal nerve

rectum posteriorly, forming a sling. The puborectalis muscle is responsible for the anorectal angle (see The Normal Process of Defecation).

Innervation

Internal Anal Sphincter

Extrinsic autonomic fibers of both the sympathetic and parasympathetic nervous systems innervate the internal anal sphincter.

External Anal Sphincter

The pudendal nerve (sacral nerve roots S2, S3 and S4) innervates the external anal sphincter, the levator ani, and the puborectalis muscles (see Fig. 1.4).

Rectum

The rectum is innervated by the sympathetic nervous system via the pelvic plexus (L1, L2, and L3), and the parasympathetic nervous system via the nervi erigentes (S2, S3, and S4).

Vascular Supply

Anal

Arterial

The superior, middle, and inferior rectal arteries supply blood to the anus.

Venous

Internal hemorrhoidal plexus connects to the superior rectal veins, which drain into the inferior mesenteric vein, which connects to the portal venous system. *External hemorrhoidal plexus* connects to the middle rectal veins and pudendal veins, which drain into the internal iliac vein, which connects to the inferior vena cava.

Rectal

Arterial

Arterial supply to the rectum occurs via the superior rectal, middle rectal, and inferior rectal arteries (see Fig. 1.5). The superior rectal artery is a branch of the inferior mesenteric artery. The middle rectal artery originates from the internal iliac or the pudendal artery, and the inferior rectal artery originates from the internal iliac artery. The majority of the blood supply is from the superior and inferior rectal arteries.

Venous

Venous drainage of the majority of the rectum occurs via the middle rectal vein, which connects to the inferior vena cava, and the superior rectal vein, which connects to the portal vein (see Fig. 1.6).

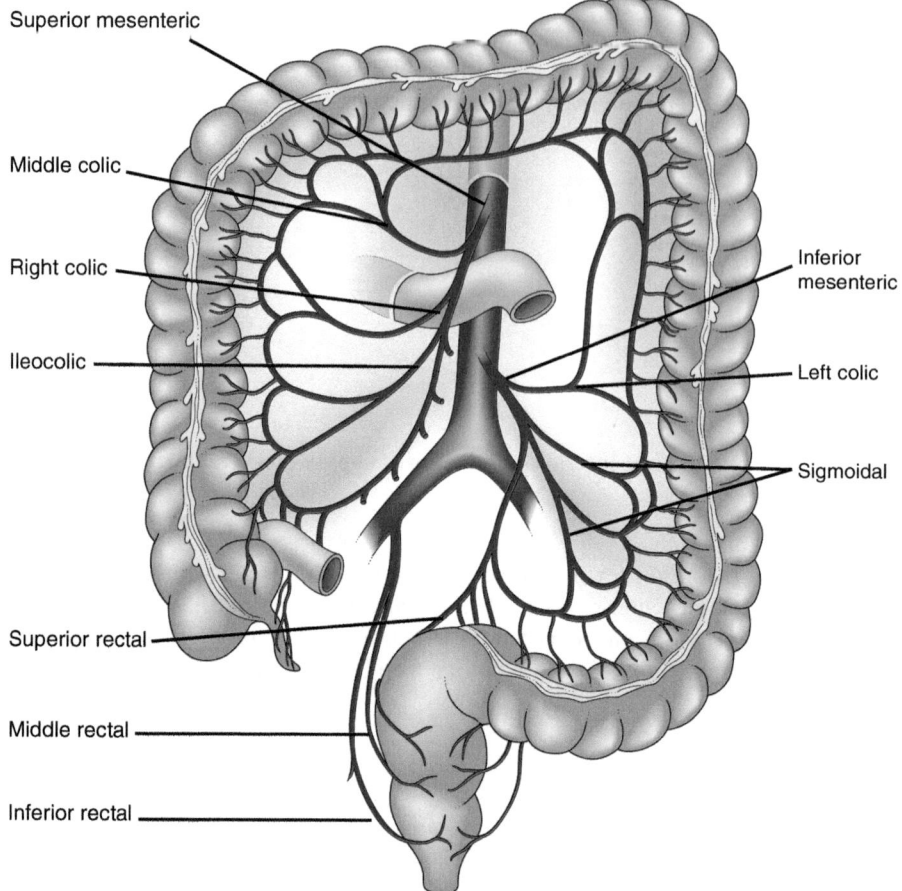

Superior mesenteric

Middle colic

Right colic

Ileocolic

Inferior mesenteric

Left colic

Sigmoidal

Superior rectal

Middle rectal

Inferior rectal

Fig. 1.5 The arterial supply to the colon originates from the superior and inferior mesenteric arteries

The Normal Process of Defecation

The neuromuscular anatomy of the anus and rectum is "designed" to preserve fecal continence and to facilitate defecation: withholding stool until it is appropriate to defecate and propelling stool at the time of defecation. The puborectalis muscle remains tonically contracted at rest to form the anorectal angle, a sharp angulation (normally approximately 90 degrees), which blocks stool from exiting out of the rectum (see Figs. 1.7 and 1.8). The anal sphincters further function to provide a barrier for the passage of air, fluid, or solid stool to exit out of the anal canal.

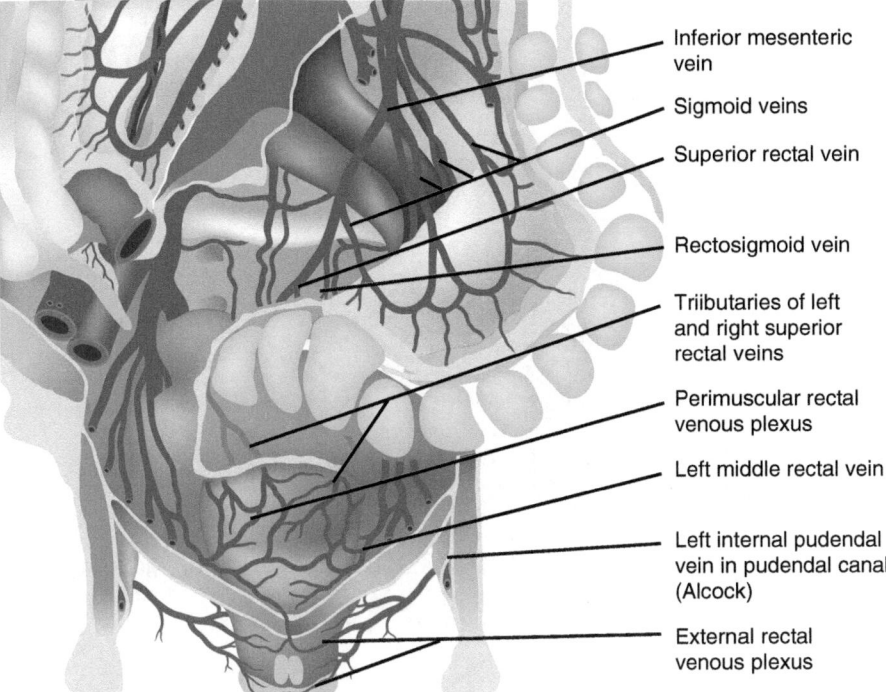

Fig. 1.6 Rectal venous anatomy

When stool enters the rectum (which is a highly compliant organ), it distends and the internal anal sphincter (which is normally contracted) relaxes, while the external anal sphincter remains closed. This process is called the rectoanal inhibitory reflex and is defective in Hirschsprung's disease. When stool is present in the rectum but defecation is not to be initiated, the puborectalis muscle and external anal sphincter remain contracted. At the appropriate time for defecation, the puborectalis muscle relaxes and the anorectal angle increases, contraction of the diaphragm and abdominal muscles increases interabdominal pressure, relaxation of the external anal sphincter occurs, and feces are passed in conjunction with contraction of the rectum (see Fig. 1.9). Increased contraction of the puborectalis muscle and external anal sphincter will occur when there is sensation of stool within the anal canal and voluntary defecation has not been initiated.

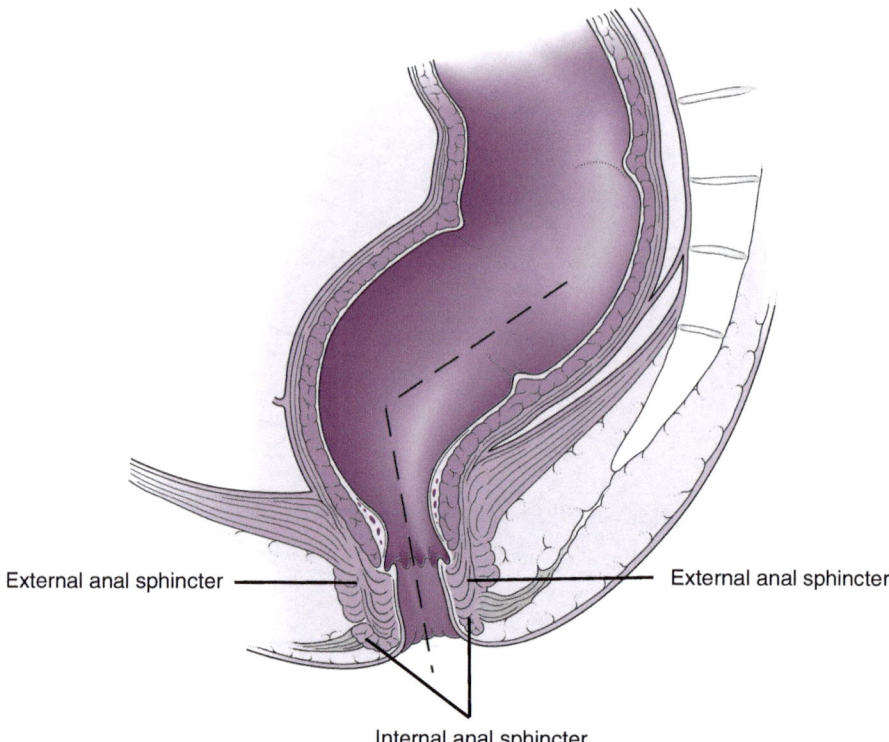

External anal sphincter ————

External anal sphincter

Internal anal sphincter

Fig. 1.7 The pull of the puborectalis anteriorly towards the pubis muscle contributes to the angulation between the rectum and anal canal termed "anorectal angle" (*dashed line*)

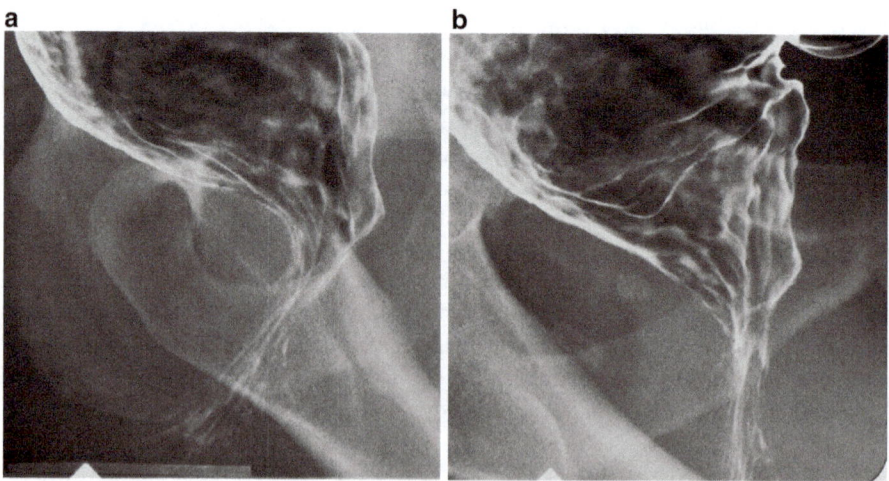

Fig. 1.8 Normal dynamic proctogram (**a**) at rest and (**b**) straining demonstrating straightening of the anorectal angle

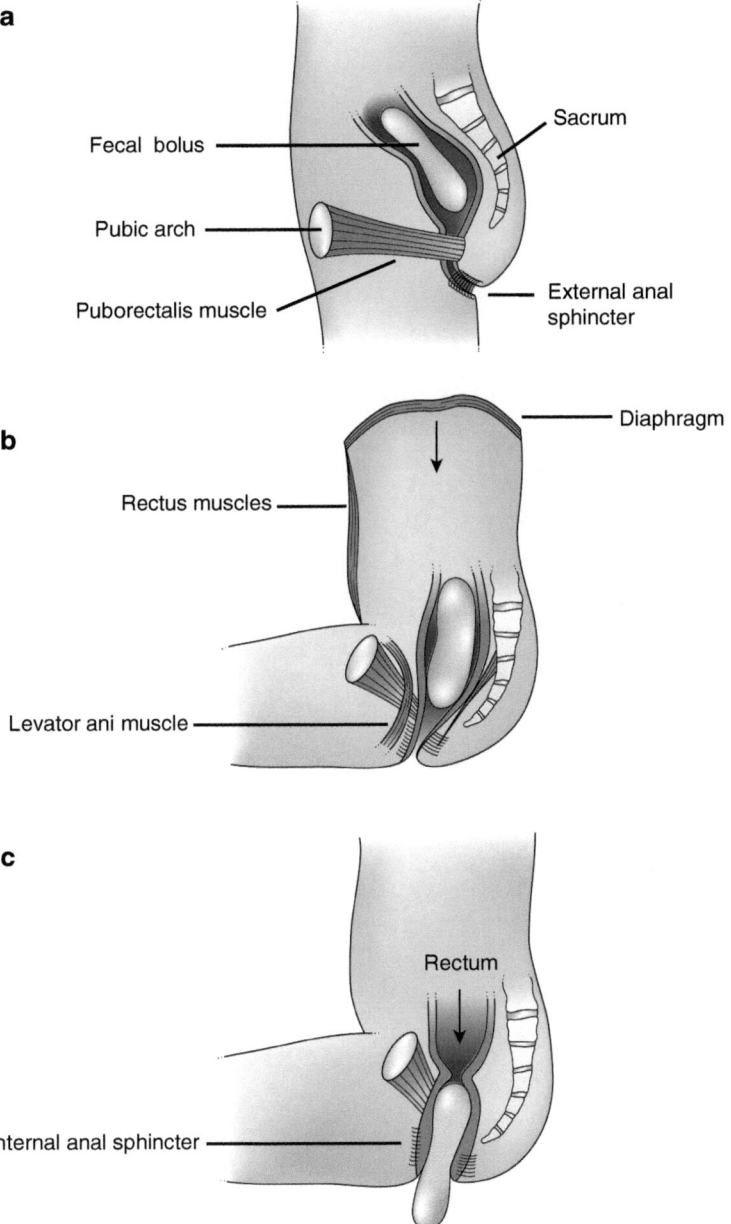

Fig. 1.9 The process of defecation. (**a**) Puborectalis and external sphincter are contracted at rest. (**b**) With entry of the stool into the rectum, the puborectalis and anal sphincters relax; the levatorani, rectus muscles, and diaphragm contract. (**c**) With defecation, the external anal sphincter relaxes; there is a rectal contraction

Chapter 2
Diagnostic Procedures

Eli D. Ehrenpreis

Anorectal Manometry

Description of Procedure

Anorectal manometry is widely used to diagnose abnormalities of anorectal function. This test employs a pressure-sensitive catheter connected to a transducer. The catheter device is inserted into the anus, and anal pressure is measured throughout the length of the anal canal. The transducer translates the mechanical pressures into an electrical signal, which is converted to a computerized readout and used to interpret the data obtained.

Indications

Chronic constipation, fecal incontinence, documentation of the presence or absence of rectoanal inhibitory reflex (RAIR) for the diagnosis of Hirschsprung's disease (see Fig. 2.1), and preoperative use prior to ileoanal pouch or colorectal anastomosis. Anorectal manometry can also be used as an adjunctive tool for performance of anorectal biofeedback.

E.D. Ehrenpreis, MD (✉)
Chief of Gastroenterology and Endoscopy, Highland Park Hospital,
NorthShore University Health System, Highland Park, IL 60035, USA

Clinical Associate Professor of Medicine, University of Chicago Medical Center,
Highland Park, IL 60035, USA
e-mail: ehrenpreis@gipharm.net

E.D. Ehrenpreis et al. (eds.), *Anal and Rectal Diseases: A Concise Manual*,
DOI 10.1007/978-1-4614-1102-4_2, © Springer Science+Business Media, LLC 2012

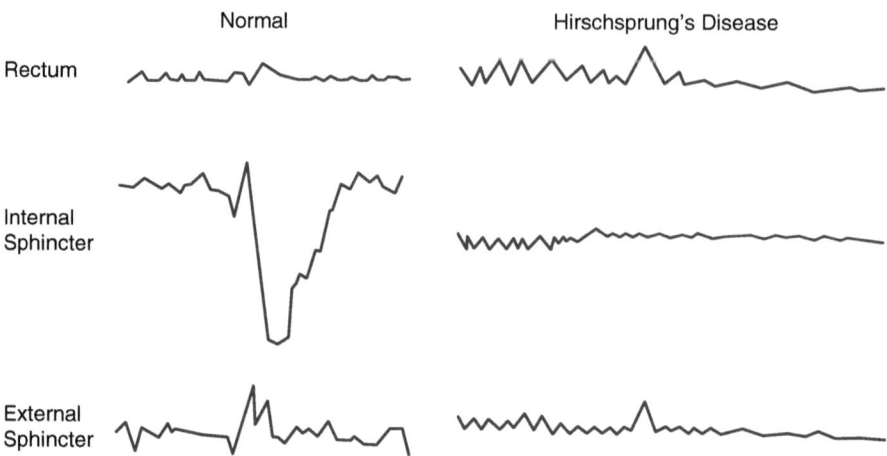

Fig. 2.1 The RAIR demonstrated in a normal subject and absent in a patient with Hirschsprung's disease

Complementary Procedures

Dynamic proctography, anorectal electromyography (EMG) and pudendal nerve terminal motor latency (PNTML) study, flexible sigmoidoscopy, full-thickness biopsy of the rectum (for diagnosis of Hirschsprung's disease), and anorectal ultrasound.

Contraindications

Anal obstruction.

Relative Contraindications

Severe anal pain and anal stricture.

Preparation of Patient

The patient should receive one or two cleansing enemas several hours prior to examination. You should also talk with them prior to the procedure to answer any concerns they may have so that they are relaxed and cooperative when the procedure begins.

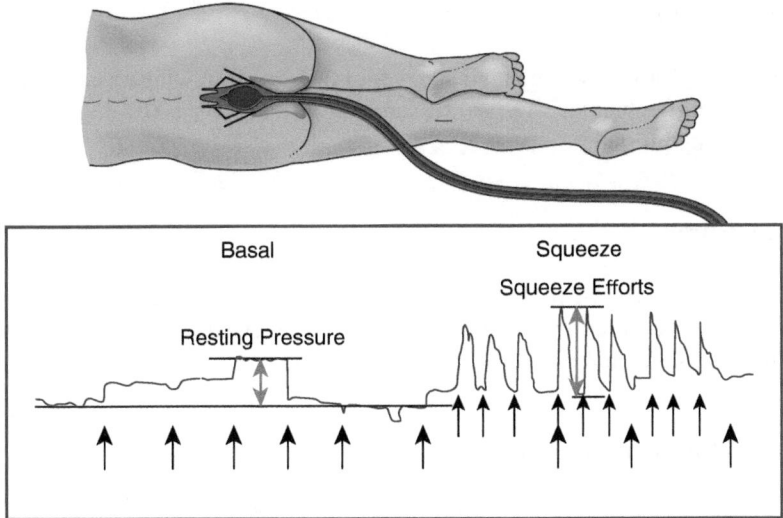

Fig. 2.2 Demonstration of the HPZ and resting and squeeze pressures using a pull-through technique

How the Procedure Is Performed

The patient is placed in a left lateral position with flexion of the knees and hips, and proper draping for adequate modesty. Pressure-sensitive catheters (balloon system, water perfusion system, or solid-state microtransducer system) are gently placed in the anal canal following calibration of the manometer. The pressure is measured through eight channels placed around the catheter, each 1 cm apart and extending 5 cm from the distal portion of the catheter. The pressure in each channel is generally measured with a "pull-through technique" (the probe is placed in the rectum and gradually withdrawn) (see Fig. 2.2). The pressure readings obtained provide a longitudinal pressure profile of the anal sphincter. The parameters measured are discussed in the following sections.

High-Pressure Zone

The high-pressure zone (HPZ) is usually present 1–1.5 cm proximal to the anal verge. This is a portion of the anal canal where pressures are greater than 50% above the average pressures within the remainder of the anal canal.

Resting Pressure

Resting pressure is measured at the HPZ. The average value is 65–85 mmHg.

Squeeze Pressure

The patient performs a squeezing maneuver of the anus following an explanation by the performing technician. These pressures are usually 50–100% higher than the average resting pressure.

Push Pressure

The patient is instructed to perform the push maneuver, mimicking an attempt to defecate. The measured pressure tracings are then viewed to determine whether a normal decrease in anal pressure occurs.

Rectoanal Inhibitory Reflex

Following the above maneuvers, a latex balloon is placed over the manometry catheter, which is then repositioned 2 cm from the anal verge. Small volumes of air are introduced into the balloon (typically beginning with 40 mL). Baseline resting anal pressures are measured to determine whether resting pressures decrease following inflation of the balloon. This decrease in sphincter pressure is called "RAIR." If no reflex is detected, the balloon is deflated and reinflated at a higher volume, such as 60 mL. Volumes of up to 180 mL may be required to document the presence of RAIR.

Detection of Rectal Sensation

The aforementioned balloon inflation using air or water at room temperature is performed and utilized to determine (1) the volume required to elicit an initial sensation, (2) the volume required to produce a sensation of urgency, and (3) the maximum tolerable volume. Volumes of up to 300 mL may be utilized to determine rectal volume sensation.

Pressure measurements may be used to map the symmetry of the anal sphincter. The presence of marked anal asymmetry is seen with sphincter damage or other abnormalities.

Changes in pressure with balloon inflation at different volumes may be used to determine rectal compliance. These studies are generally used for research purposes. Rectal compliance measurements have been used to show, for example, that some patients with irritable bowel syndrome have decreased rectal compliance, enhancing the sense of urgency experienced in the condition.

Typical Abnormal Findings

The most common abnormal findings on anorectal manometry and the possible causes of these abnormalities are shown in Table 2.1.

Table 2.1 Common abnormal findings on anorectal manometry and their possible causes

Finding	Cause
Elevated resting pressure	Anal sphincter spasm (anismus), nonrelaxing puborectalis syndrome, hemorrhoids, anal fissure
Decreased resting and squeeze pressures	Anal injury secondary to trauma, anal surgery or obstetric injury, neurologic diseases, or anorectal prolapse
Absence of the fall in resting anal pressure with push maneuver	Anismus or nonrelaxing puborectalis syndrome
Absence or RAIR	Hirschsprung's disease or megacolon/megarectum
Lowered threshold of rectal sensation	Irritable bowel syndrome or post-gastroenteritis hypersensitivity
Decreased rectal sensation	Altered sensorium, central nervous system disease, neurologic disorders, or megacolon/megarectum
Decrease rectal compliance	Colitis, radiation proctopathy, or irritable bowel syndrome

Complications

None.

Additional Comments

Biofeedback techniques have been successfully utilized in conjunction with anorectal manometry to assist with retraining of the anal sphincter in patients with fecal incontinence and spastic anorectal disorders.

Anoscopy and Proctoscopy

Description of Procedure

Anoscopy (endoscopic examination of anal mucosa and lower rectum) and proctoscopy (endoscopic examination of entire rectum) involve the placement of a rigid plastic or metal instrument (anoscope/proctoscope – see Fig. 2.3) into the anal canal. The proctoscope has either an internal or external light source.

Indications

Anal pain, discharge, rectal bleeding, internal or external hemorrhoids, pruritus ani, palpable mass on digital rectal examination, or anal condyloma.

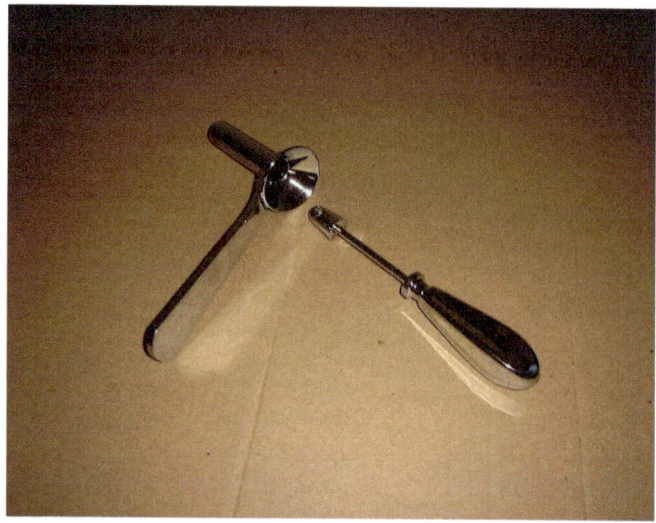

Fig. 2.3 A Naunton Morgan proctoscope (image courtesy of B and H Surgical Instrument Makers, London, UK)

Complementary Procedures

Flexible sigmoidoscopy and colonoscopy.

Contraindications

Acute myocardial infarction (due to the potential of inducing a vagal response) and a patient who is unable/unwilling to cooperate with the procedure.

Relative Contraindications

Suspected acute abdomen, debilitated patient, or anal stenosis.

Preparation of Patient

Patient reassurance is mandatory. Generally, no preparation is required for the procedure, although an enema may be used if necessary.

How the Procedure Is Performed

The patient is placed in a left lateral position. A local anesthetic may be applied to the anal region. A digital examination is performed after lubrication of the gloved finger. The anoscope or proctoscope is lubricated and placed gently into the anus. This is advanced slowly following relaxation of the anal sphincter. Sometimes, gentle rotation of the device eases insertion. After full advancement of the scope, the inner obturator is removed. Suctioning may be performed to clear the view, and a light source is utilized to obtain good visualization. The scope is gently withdrawn for evaluation, and the walls of the anus and rectum are viewed. Biopsies and suctioning of fecal material for culture and microscopy may be performed.

Typical Abnormal Findings

Anal or rectal lesions such as hemorrhoids or neoplasms. Biopsies of lesions may be obtained, and suctioned material collected for culture and microscopic evaluation. The collected material is useful for diagnosing sexually transmitted diseases of the anus and rectum.

Complications

Patient discomfort and/or embarrassment are common. Uncommon complications include tearing of the anoderm or postbiopsy bleeding.

Additional Comments

Anoscopy and proctoscopy have been replaced by flexible sigmoidoscopy in many clinical practices.

Barium Enema

Description of Procedure

A barium enema is a radiographic examination of the colon (see Fig. 2.4a, b). It is performed using either a single column of barium sulfate instilled into the colon or a barium instillation combined with air to perform an air-contrast study.

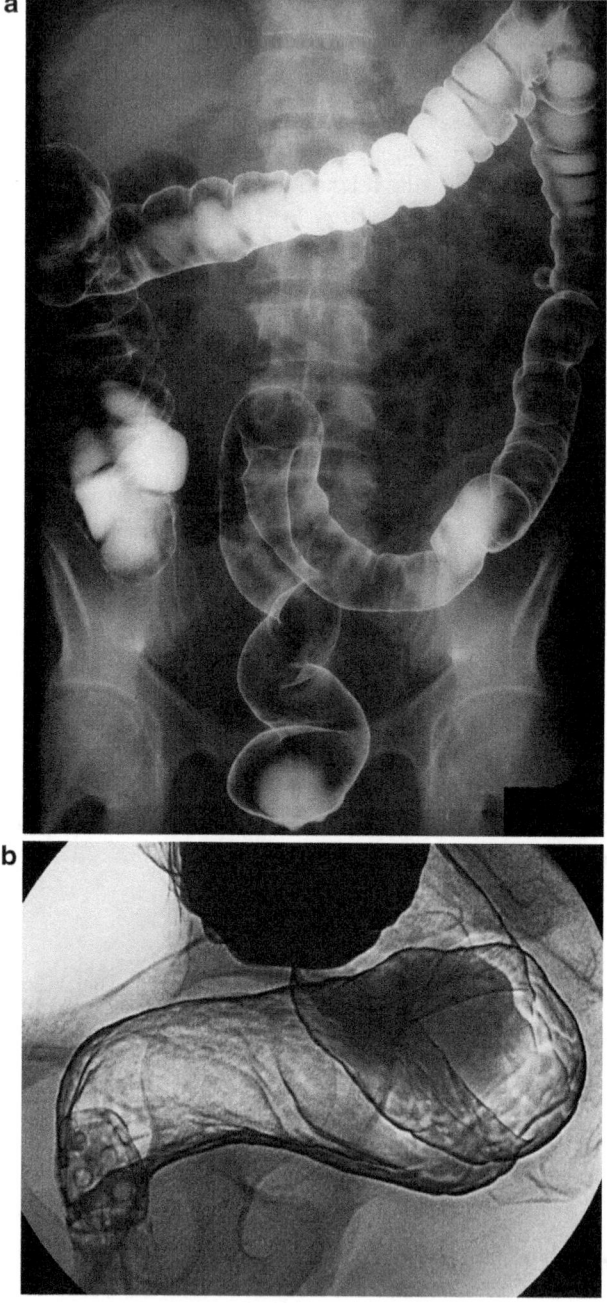

Fig. 2.4 (a) Normal view of the colon on barium enema examination. A single diverticulum is noted in the descending colon (*arrow*). (b) Normal view of the rectum on barium enema. Enema tip is present

Indications

Evaluation of symptoms suggestive of colonic disease, such as constipation, rectal bleeding, irritable bowel syndrome, and unexplained diarrhea. Complete evaluation of the colon for colorectal cancer screening or surveillance when colonoscopy is contraindicated or cannot be safely or adequately performed.

Complementary Procedures

Colonoscopy, anorectal manometry, EMG, defecography, abdominal and pelvic computed tomography (CT) scan, stool culture, stool microscopy, stool for *Clostridium difficile* toxin testing, fecal fat testing, and electrolyte examination.

Contraindications

Prior allergic reaction to barium, imperforate anus, bowel obstruction, or tight stricture of the colon.

Relative Contraindications

Inability to prepare a patient, a patient who is unwilling or unable to cooperate with the procedure, or a colonic stricture.

Preparation of Patient

This usually takes place over 2 days. On day 1, patients begin a low residue diet with encouragement of liquid intake. On day 2, patients initiate a clear liquid diet. This is complemented by administration of laxatives, enemas, and/or suppositories. In our practice, patients are encouraged to drink one 8 oz bottle of magnesium citrate at 12:00 (midday) on day 2. This is followed by two bisacodyl tablets at 16:00 and 20:00. Clear liquids are encouraged until 22:00, after which no further intake of food or liquids is allowed. At 06:00 on the day of the study, the patient self-administers one bisacodyl suppository.

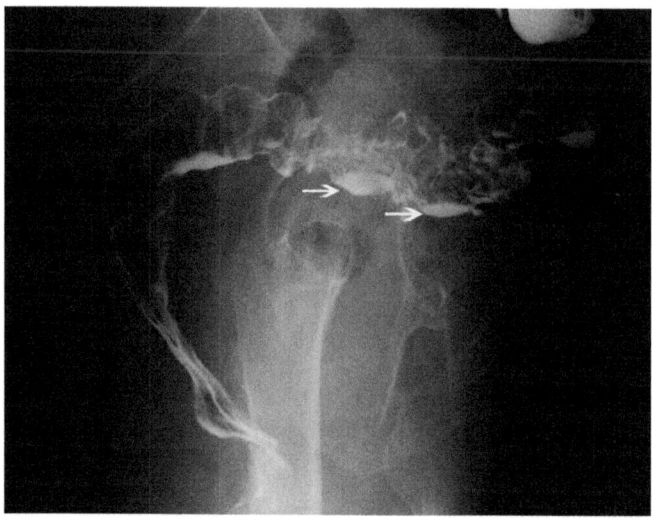

Fig. 2.5 Marked sigmoid diverticulosis (*arrows*) demonstrated on barium enema. The colon is poorly distensible

How the Procedure Is Performed

The technician places a catheter into the rectum and barium is injected to fill the colon. Intravenous glucagon is often administered to assist with distribution of the barium. Barium placed into the colon provides contrast material to outline colonic lesions and makes them visible on X-ray films. Fluoroscopy is used (with the patient in a supine position) to visualize the posterior portions of the colon, and with the patient in a prone position to evaluate the anterior colonic walls. Patients are turned periodically to coat the entire colon with barium. Subsequently, air is instilled to provide air contrast by spreading the barium into a thin layer along the colonic wall. A balloon is placed and inflated in the rectum to prevent discharge of the barium. During the procedure, fluoroscopy and static X-rays are obtained at various angles to visualize all regions of the colon. After evacuation of the barium, the images of the colon are examined for mucosal abnormalities and anatomic disruptions.

Typical Abnormal Findings

Alterations of colonic anatomy such as tortuosity and increased length of the sigmoid colon in chronic constipation or loss of haustration in cases of laxative abuse may be identified. The barium enema may reveal causes of constipation, abdominal or pelvic pain, and diarrhea, such as obstructing colonic lesions, severe diverticular disease (see Fig. 2.5), ulcerative colitis, and Crohn's disease.

Complications

Barium enemas are usually very well tolerated, although discomfort and embarrassment are common during the procedure. Perforation, dehydration, barium concretion, severe constipation, and obstipation are relatively rare.

Additional Comments

Barium enema examination will miss up to 10% of colorectal cancers and colonic polyps and is therefore not recommended as a first-line procedure for colorectal cancer screening or surveillance. The inflated rectal balloon that is present during the performance of the barium enema limits visualization of the rectum; therefore, a proctoscopy or sigmoidoscopy is required for complete colonic evaluation. Barium enemas may be combined with defecography in a single test for constipation. This combined test is used in patients with chronic constipation to rule out anatomic abnormalities and to evaluate for the presence of pelvic floor disorders.

Biofeedback Therapy

Description of Procedure

Biofeedback therapy is a form of pelvic muscular retraining.

Indications

Chronic constipation and fecal incontinence.

Complementary Procedures

Kegel exercises, defecography, balloon expulsion testing, testing of rectal sensation, and intrasphincteric botulinum toxin (Botox) injections.

Contraindications

Imperforate anus.

Relative Contraindications

Inability of the patient to understand or cooperate with the procedure.

Preparation of Patient

Some centers recommend that patients use two Cleansing enemas on the morning of the procedure: others perform the procedure without preparation with Fleet's enemas.

How the Procedure Is Performed

Anal EMG or anorectal manometry is used to provide biofeedback during pelvic retraining. Exercises are generally performed for 1 h/week. Initially, patients are educated on the function of the pelvic floor muscles, often with the use of a video demonstration. This increases patient understanding and compliance, and encourages patient participation in the procedure. Patients are then taught to appreciate the difference in sensation between anal resting, squeezing, and pushing. Measurements of anal pressures and activity during these maneuvers are obtained using anorectal manometry or EMG. Patients perform Kegel exercises and relaxation techniques at home and chart home bowel activities. Follow-up sessions with manometry or EMG measurements are performed. Biofeedback therapists use reinforcement techniques and set specific objective goals (based on manometric or EMG measurements) for resting, pushing, and squeezing maneuvers. Biofeedback therapists may utilize additional techniques during the sessions to assist patients in stress management, proper bathroom goals, and lifestyle modification.

Results Obtained

A number of studies have demonstrated that biofeedback therapy is highly successful for the treatment of pelvic floor-related defecation disorders (84% of patients undergoing the procedure report improvement in their symptoms). This technique is also relatively successful in patients with fecal incontinence.

Complications

There are no complications per se; the technique is usually well tolerated, although mild discomfort may occur.

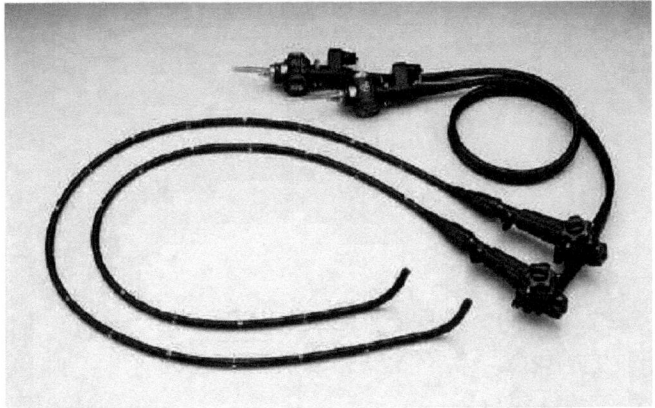

Fig. 2.6   A colonoscopy (CF240-DLI, courtesy of KeyMed Ltd)

Additional Comments

Biofeedback therapy has also been utilized for the treatment of other forms of chronic constipation and for irritable bowel syndrome.

Colonoscopy

Description of Procedure

A colonoscopy is an endoscopic investigation of the colon using a colonoscope; a flexible device that is 8–12 mm in diameter and 120–230 cm in length (see Fig. 2.6). It is inserted into the anal canal and advanced proximally to the cecum (and at times to the terminal ileum) (see Fig. 2.7). The colonoscope provides a well-lit, magnified view of the colonic mucosa. It has a suction channel to remove fecal material for analysis and a biopsy port to obtain mucosal specimens for histologic evaluation. Hemostasis of bleeding lesions can be performed through this channel using injection therapy with epinephrine and thermal coagulation therapy.

Indications

Evaluation of an abnormality seen on barium enema, gastrointestinal bleeding, unexplained iron deficiency anemia, surveillance of patients with a history of colon cancer or colonic polyps, screening of high-risk individuals for colon cancer or

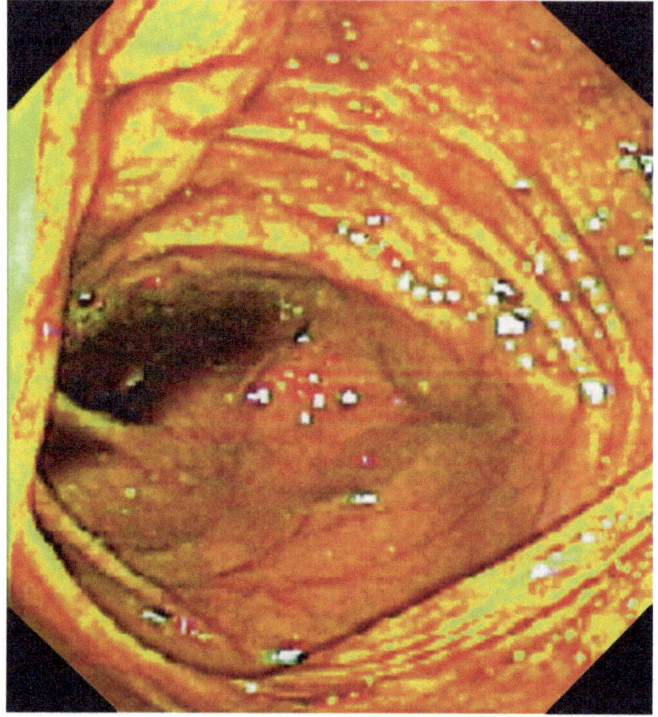

Fig. 2.7 The base of the cecum and ileocecal valve demonstrated on colonoscopy

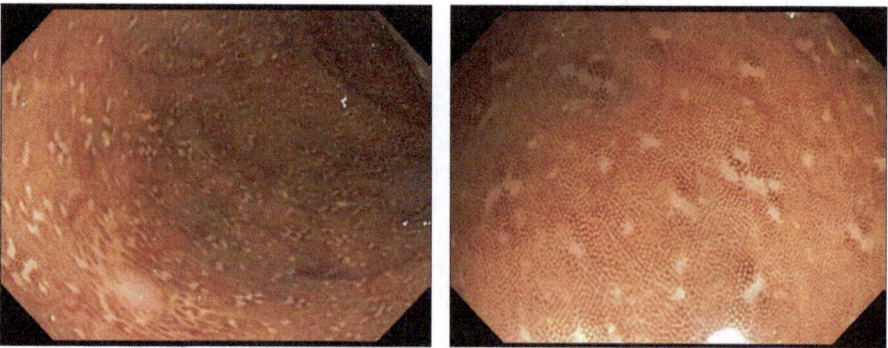

Fig. 2.8 Melanosis coli of the colonic mucosa seen during colonoscopy. The mucosa has a speckled or snake skin appearance. Pale areas represent sparing of lymphoid aggregates. Lipfuscin accumulation in histiocytes causes the characteristic darkening of the mucosa

colonic polyps, screening of normal individuals for colon cancer or colonic polyps, evaluation of patients with chronic inflammatory bowel disease or unexplained diarrhea, other mucosal abnormalities (see Fig. 2.8), and intraoperative evaluation of colonic lesions.

Complementary Procedures

Small intestine radiography, upper endoscopy, and CT scan of the abdomen and pelvis.

Contraindications

Fulminant colitis, acute severe diverticulitis, and suspected gastrointestinal perforation.

Relative Contraindications

Inability to prepare for the procedure (since the colon must be purged for a complete evaluation), inability to obtain consent for the procedure, lack of intravenous access, inability to provide adequate sedation to complete examination, and coagulopathy.

Preparation of Patient

This generally begins the day prior to the procedure. A clear liquid diet is started in the afternoon before the colonoscopy. On the evening before and then morning of the procedure, the patient should consume 1–2 liters of polyethylene glycol in a balanced electrolyte solution over 2–5 h. An oral sodium phosphate preparation in tablet form has been introduced. Lower volume preparations are available.

How the Procedure Is Performed

The patient is usually placed in a left lateral position. Intravenous sedation (usually combining an opioid such as meperidine and a benzodiazepine such as midazolam or diazepam) is administered. A digital rectal examination is performed. The colonoscope is introduced and advanced to the cecum. External pressure and position changes are often required to allow a safe, full evaluation of the colon. If Crohn's disease is suspected, or a more proximal source of gastrointestinal bleeding is considered, the ileocecal valve is traversed and the colonoscope is introduced into the terminal ileum. After confirmation of the location of the tip of the colonoscope in the cecum, the scope is gradually withdrawn.

Any polyps that are seen on colonoscope withdrawal are removed. Techniques for polyp removal include snaring the polyp with or without electrocautery and performance of a biopsy with associated electrocautery. Multiple biopsies are performed on suspected cancers or lesions that are too large to remove with the colonoscope. If patients are evaluated for unexplained diarrhea, biopsies of the colon (and sometimes the ileum) are obtained in abnormal as well as apparently normal mucosa. In patients with ulcerative colitis or Crohn's disease who are receiving colonoscopic surveillance, biopsies are obtained from each of the four quadrants every 10 cm for histologic evaluation to rule out dysplasia. Retroflexion of the colonoscope in the distal rectum allows visualization of the proximal anal canal and the dentate line. This is particularly useful when looking for internal hemorrhoids and distal rectal or high anal canal lesions. The retroflexed view is also useful for finding and removing polyps in the distal rectum.

Typical Abnormal Findings

Full evaluation of the colonic mucosa is obtained with colonoscopy. Identification and removal of colonic polyps is performed (see Figs. 2.9–2.11). Identification of sources of colonic bleeding (see Figs. 2.12 and 2.13), evaluation of the distal rectum and anal canal for bleeding sources, diagnosis of inflammatory bowel disease, determination of endoscopic and histologic severity of inflammatory bowel disease, surveillance of those carrying the diagnosis of ulcerative colitis or Crohn's disease, and diagnosis of microscopic colitis.

Complications

The perforation rate for colonoscopy is estimated to be between 0.2 and 1.0% (depending on whether a polypectomy has been performed). Postpolypectomy bleeding ranges from 0.4 to 2%. Dehydration and electrolyte abnormalities – including hypernatremia, hyponatremia, hypokalemia, and hypomagnesemia – may occur with sodium phosphate-based colonoscopy preparations. Several cases of severe hyponatremia have been described after polyethylene glycol preparation. Respiratory depression, hypotension, and bradycardia associated with excessive sedation are infrequent. Patients may generally experience some discomfort during the procedure.

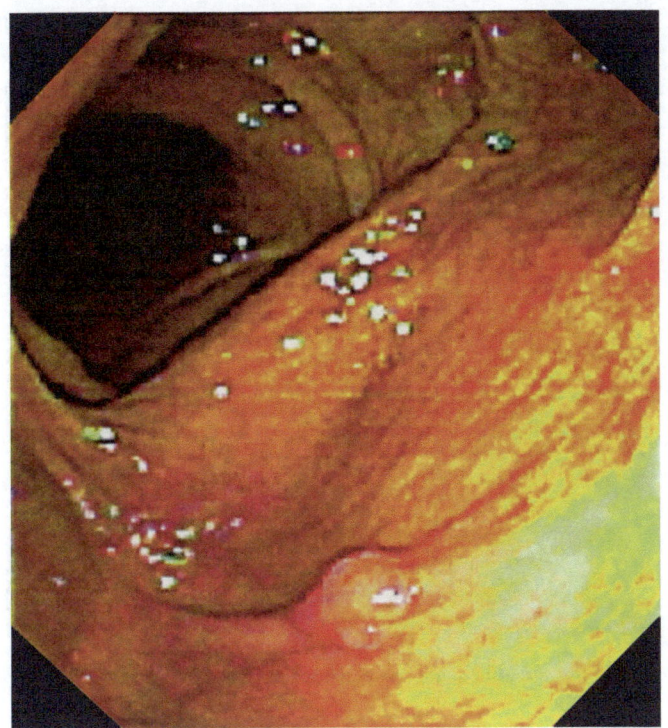

Fig. 2.9 A sessile polyp of the ascending colon

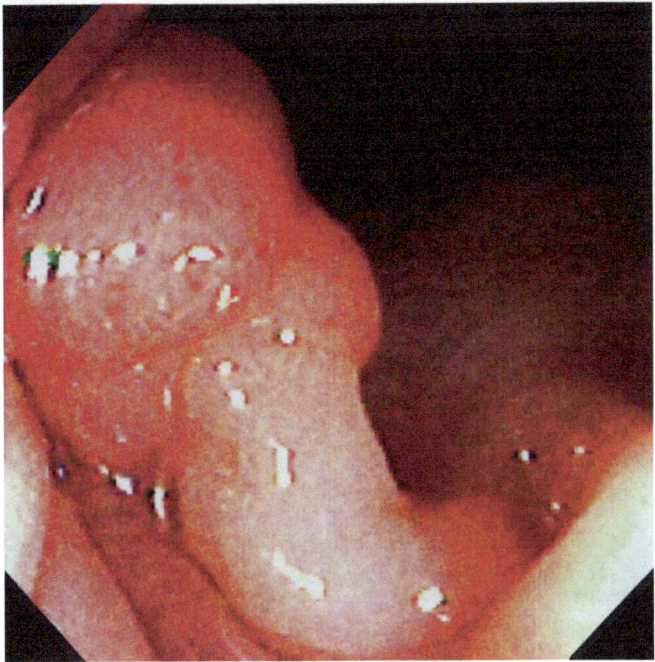

Fig. 2.10 A pedunculated polyp in the descending colon

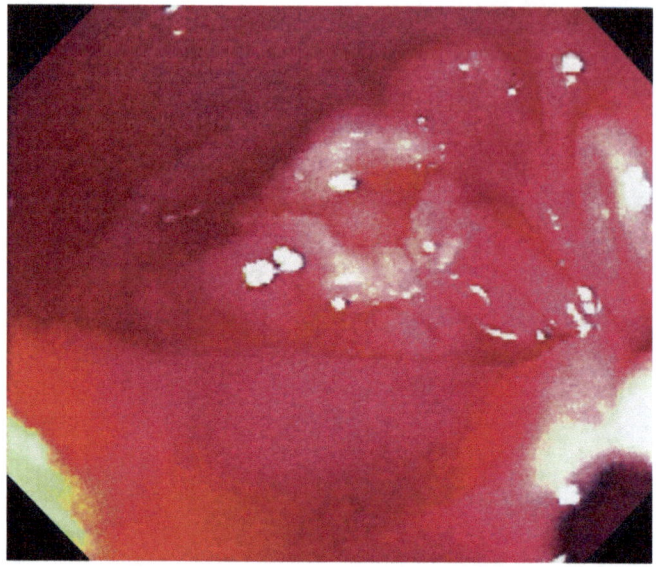

Fig. 2.11 Polypectomy site after snare and electrocautery of a polyp

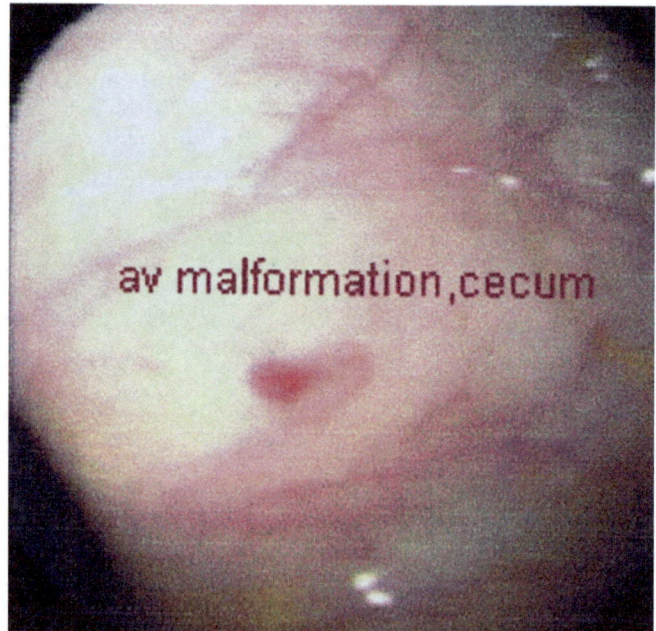

Fig. 2.12 Cecal arteriovenous malformations

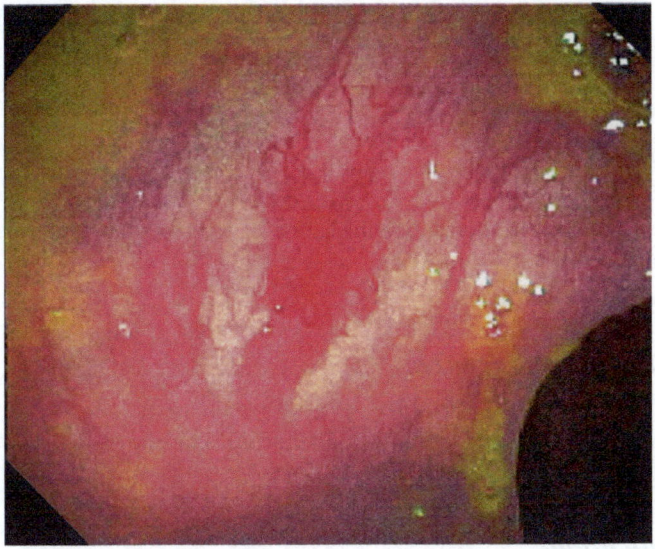

Fig. 2.13 Arteriovenous malformation of ascending colon

Additional Comments

New techniques for colon cancer screening, including CT of the colon (virtual colonoscopy) and molecular biology-based stool testing, are under investigation.

Dynamic Proctography

Description of Procedure

A small quantity (about 250 mL) of high viscosity barium is placed in the rectum. Subjects are then seated on a radiolucent commode. Lateral fluoroscopy is performed following identification of the anal canal. The radiologist instructs the patient to hold the barium to allow films to be taken at rest, and to squeeze the anus shut to hold in the barium to obtain "squeeze" films. Finally, the patient is asked to strain and attempt to evacuate the barium. Continuous video fluoroscopy is the preferred method of obtaining data. Static views are also obtained, and the anatomic position of the pubococcygeal line is determined. Lateral films are utilized to measure the anorectal angle between the anal canal and the horizontal axis of the rectum (located approximately 2 cm above the ischial tuberosity). This technique can identify changes in the anorectal angle, alteration of anorectal anatomy, and abnormal mobility of the pelvic floor with the aforementioned maneuvers

Indications

Constipation, fecal incontinence, identification of rectovaginal fistulas, and evaluation of ileoanal pouch anastomoses.

Complementary Procedures

Barium enema, EMG, anorectal ultrasound, and colonoscopy.

Contraindications

Allergy to barium, imperforate anus, or tight rectal stricture.

Relative Contraindications

Inability of the patient to cooperate with the procedure.

Preparation of Patient

Most radiologists recommend colonic cleansing using a saline-based cathartic laxative such as magnesium citrate and/or enemas. A few perform the procedure without prior preparation.

How the Procedure Is Performed

As described earlier, analysis of static and dynamic data is required. In normal patients, the anorectal angle is approximately 90° at rest, increasing to >135° with straining and defecation, and decreasing to about 75° with squeeze maneuvers (see Figs. 2.14 and 2.15). The presence of a widened resting anorectal angle can be seen in patients with neurogenic incontinence. Abnormalities such as rectoceles and anorectal intussusception can also be determined during maneuvers.

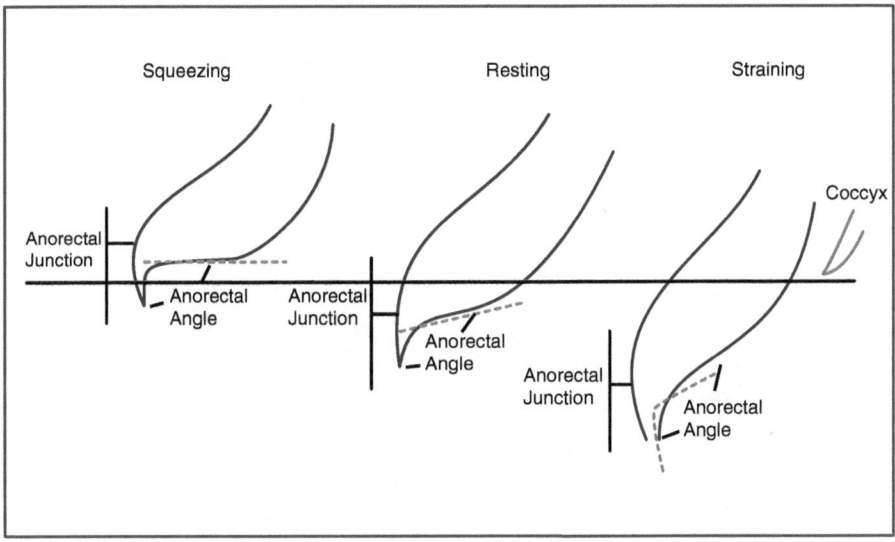

Fig. 2.14 Normal changes of the anorectal angle and anal canal seen with maneuvers during dynamic proctography

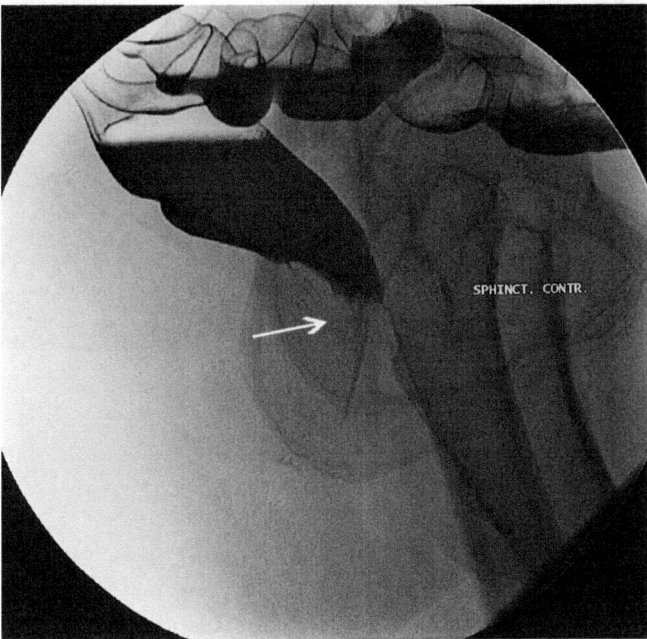

Fig. 2.15 Squeeze maneuver on dynamic proctography. Barium does not move into the anal canal due to comtraction of the puborectalis muscle (*arrow*)

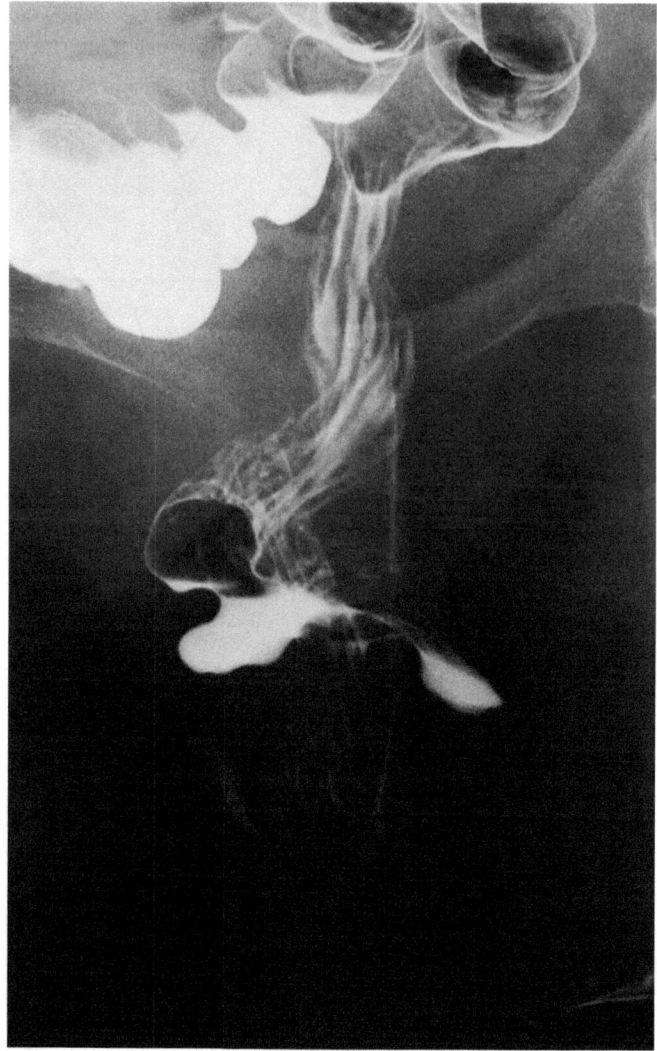

Fig. 2.16 Lateral rectoceles demonstrated on dynamic proctography

Typical Abnormal Findings

Dynamic proctography may reveal abnormalities as described earlier. Alterations in the anorectal angle can be seen, and nonrelaxing puborectalis syndrome or anismus can be diagnosed. Rectocele (see Fig. 2.16), abnormal pelvic descent, anorectal intussusception, anovaginal fistula (see Fig. 2.17), pubococcygeal tear (see Fig. 2.18), ileoanal pouch leakage, and rectal prolapse may all be diagnosed.

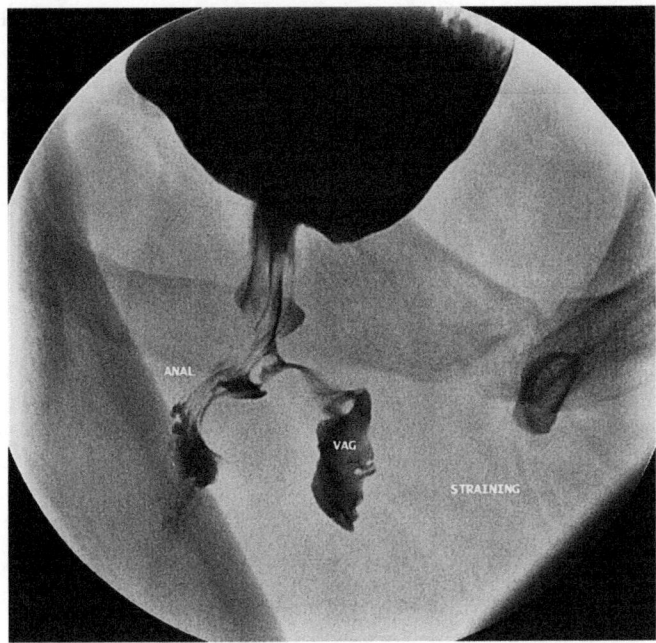

Fig. 2.17 Oblique view of an anovaginal fistula seen on dynamic proctography

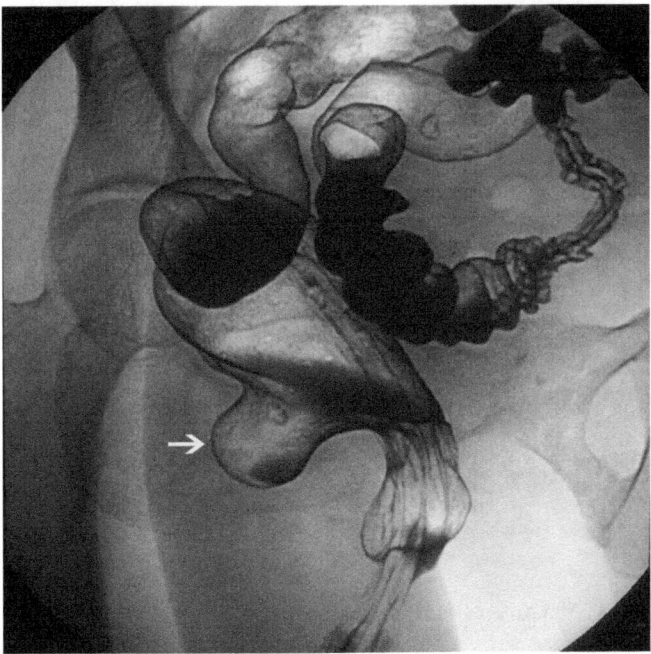

Fig. 2.18 Pubococcygeal tear with herniation of rectal tissue (*arrow*) demonstrated on dynamic proctography. Hernia was only seen when the patient bore down with contrast in place during dynamic study

Complications

Patient discomfort and barium impaction.

Additional Comments

Dynamic proctography should be performed in a center where the staff have experience with the procedure. It is a time-consuming technique and the patient must be reassured and given clear instructions during the procedure to allow for optimal cooperation. Patient embarrassment during the procedure can produce radiographic changes mimicking nonrelaxing puborectalis syndrome.

Electromyography

Description of Procedure

Anal EMG is the measurement of electrical activity in the anal muscle. The procedure involves placement of an electrode (using a needle, wire, or surface plug) onto the anal muscle. The electrical activity of the internal anal sphincter (IAS) and external anal sphincter (EAS) and the puborectalis muscles is then measured. Electrical action is measured at rest and during various maneuvers, including squeezing, pushing, and coughing (see Fig. 2.19). The signal is transferred from the record electrode to an amplifier and oscilloscope. Data are converted via a computerized formula.

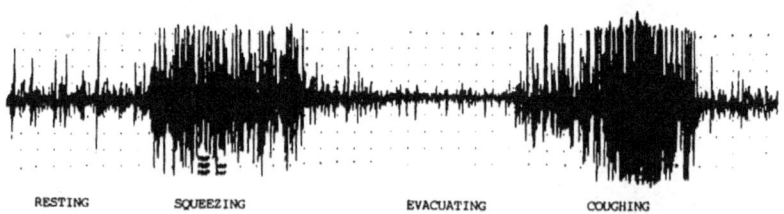

RESTING   SQUEEZING   EVACUATING   COUGHING

Fig. 2.19 Normal EMG patterns with maneuvers

Indications

Chronic constipation with suspected obstructive defecation disorders, chronic straining, suspected pelvic neuromuscular disorders, identification of anal sphincter injury, and fecal incontinence.

Complementary Procedures

Dynamic proctography, sigmoidoscopy, colonoscopy, Sitz™ marker study, anorectal ultrasound, barium enema, and PNTML.

Contraindications

Bleeding disorders or anal carcinoma.

Relative Contraindications

Inability to cooperate with testing, anal stenosis, anal abscess, or bleeding hemorrhoids.

Preparation of Patient

Some centers recommend a preparation of one or two cleansing enemas just prior to the procedure; others do not recommend any enemas as preparation for the procedure.

How the Procedure Is Performed

Catheters may consist of a needle, a small single-fiber electrode, or a small anal plug made from a plastic or sponge material upon which surface electrodes have been mounted. After application of topical anesthesia, with the patient lying in a left lateral position, EMG catheters are inserted into the IAS and EAS and puborectalis muscles. The catheters are connected to the amplifier and electrical transducer. Patients are instructed to perform various activities including squeezing, pushing (defecatory simulation), and coughing. Recordings are taken during these activities.

Typical Abnormal Findings

EMG is highly effective for diagnosing nonrelaxing puborectalis syndrome and anismus. With these abnormalities, continued or increased muscle contraction occurs during a push maneuver. In anal sphincter injuries and neuromuscular damage, decreased or erratic motor function is documented.

Complications

Patients often complain of discomfort; bleeding and/or infection are rare complications.

Additional Comments

Surface electrode techniques reduce patient discomfort and decrease the risk of infection; however, needle EMG is more accurate for documenting anal trauma and sphincter injuries. A 24-h ambulatory EMG has been proposed as a sensitive means of correlating symptoms with disorders of the anal sphincter and puborectalis muscles. Surface electrode EMG has been used in biofeedback treatment of pelvic floor disorders.

Flexible Sigmoidoscopy

Description of Procedure

Flexible sigmoidoscopes are 8–12 mm in diameter and 60 cm in length. The sigmoidoscope is inserted into the anal canal and advanced proximally as far as patient tolerance permits. The flexible sigmoidoscope provides a well-lit, magnified view of the colonic mucosa. It has a suction channel to remove fecal material for analysis and a biopsy channel to obtain mucosal specimens for histologic analysis.

Indications

Rectal bleeding, rectal mass, colitis, diarrhea, screening for colon cancer (in combination with stool Hemoccult® fecal blood testing), surveillance of patients with an ileoanal pouch, fecal incontinence (in combination with other studies), constipation (in combination with other studies), or screening of patients with a family history of familial polyposis syndromes.

Complementary Procedures

Barium enema, stool collection, Hemoccult® fecal blood test, anorectal ultrasound, anorectal manometry, and defecography.

Contraindications

Imperforate anus.

Relative Contraindications

Severe anal or rectal pain (such as that caused by an anal fissure), anal or rectal stricture, or severe coagulopathy (in which biopsies should not be performed).

Preparation of Patient

The patient should only receive clear liquids after their dinner the night or 16 h before the procedure and should be given two sodium phosphate enemas on the morning of the procedure. More aggressive preparations, such as 24 h of clear liquids and oral laxatives, have been recommended by some to improve mucosal visualization. Some clinicians recommend flexible sigmoidoscopy without preparation in patients undergoing evaluation for colitis because a preparation may alter the appearance of the mucosa.

How the Procedure Is Performed

The patient is placed in a left lateral position and a gentle digital rectal examination is performed. It is possible to perform a prostate examination on male patients at this time to screen for prostate cancer. The flexible sigmoidoscope is inserted and advanced to 60 cm, or as far as is tolerated by the patient. It is not uncommon for patient discomfort (due to sigmoid angulation and redundancy) to limit advancement of the flexible sigmoidoscope beyond 30 cm. If a large polyp is seen, the patient will undergo a colonoscopy for complete evaluation of the colon and removal of the polyp (see Fig. 2.20). If smaller polyps are seen (see Figs. 2.21 and 2.22), biopsies of these lesions are recommended. Colonoscopy is subsequently performed if adenomatous polyps are identified.

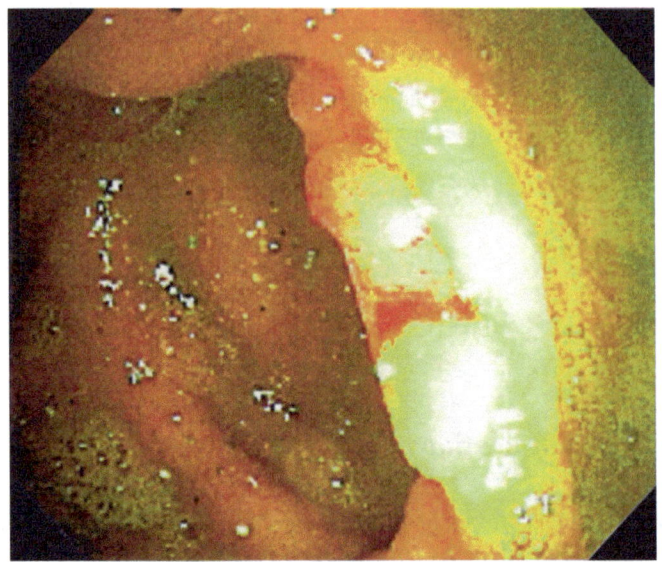

Fig. 2.20 A large sessile sigmoid polyp.

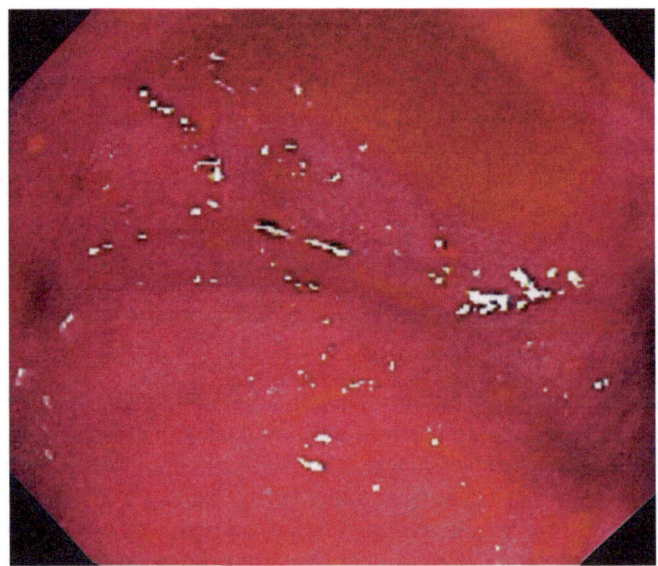

Fig. 2.21 Small sessile rectal polyp, a common finding on flexible sigmoidoscopy

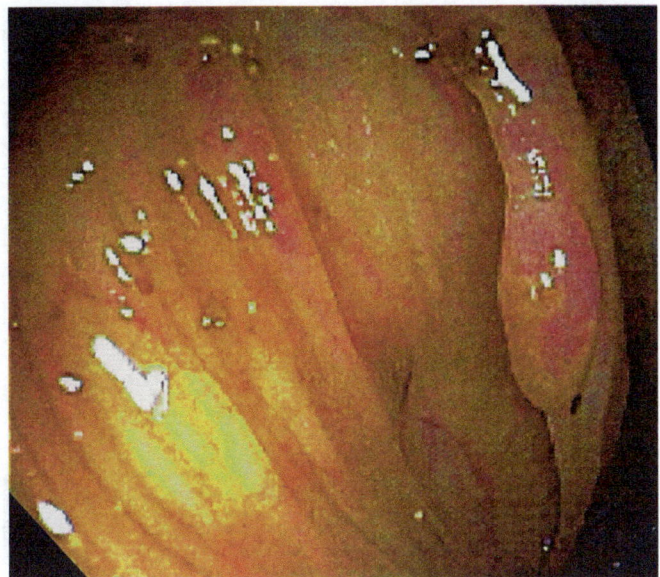

Fig. 2.22 Sigmoid colonic polyp demonstrated on flexible sigmoidoscopy

In patients with diarrhea caused by a suspected infection, fecal material may be suctioned and collected for culture, and ova, parasite, and *C. difficile* toxin PCR evaluation. Retroflexion of the sigmoidoscope in the distal rectum allows visualization of the proximal anal canal and the dentate line. This is particularly useful for looking at internal hemorrhoids and high anal canal lesions. The retroflexed view is also useful for finding polyps in the distal rectum (see Fig. 2.23). If colitis is suspected based on visualization of the mucosa and/or clinical history, biopsies are obtained and sent for histologic evaluation.

Typical Abnormal Findings

Screening of the distal 60 cm of the colon may reveal polyps or colon cancer; evaluation of the distal 60 cm of the colon allows for identification of sources of rectal bleeding, including hemorrhoids and proctocolitis. Biopsies may be obtained for suspected colitis if the mucosal appearance is abnormal. Diverticulosis of the colon may also be identified (see Fig. 2.24).

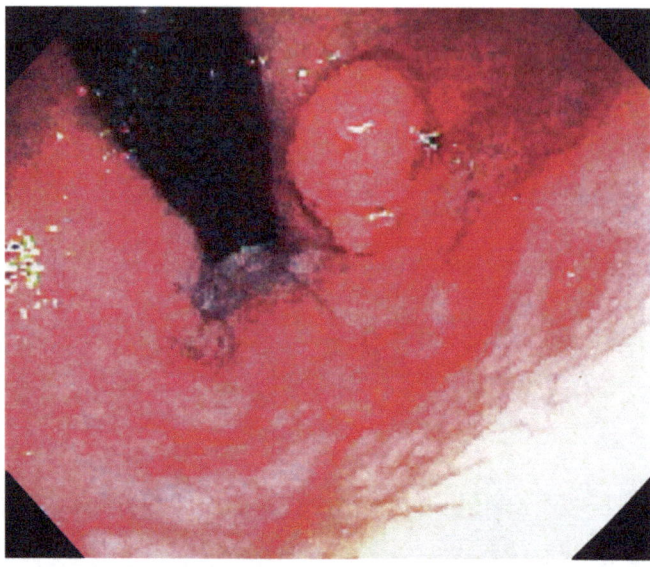

Fig. 2.23 A sessile polyp near the dentate line seen on retroflexion of the sigmoidoscope

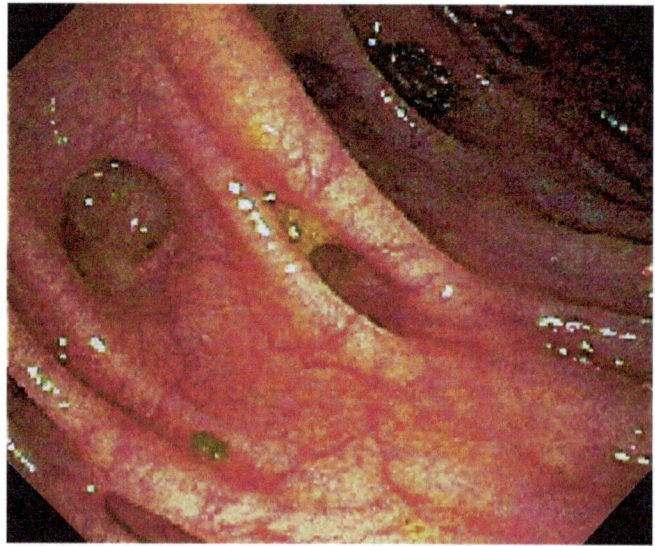

Fig. 2.24 Sigmoid diverticulosis, a common endoscopic finding

Complications

Patient discomfort is common. Bleeding may occur subsequent to biopsies. Perforation is a very rare complication of flexible sigmoidoscopy.

Additional Comments

In the United States, colonoscopy with visualization of the entire colon is replacing flexible sigmoidoscopy as the preferred method for screening for colon polyps and cancers.

Pudendal Nerve Terminal Motor Latency

Description of Procedure

The pudendal nerve innervates the anal sphincters; therefore, pudendal nerve injury may result in sphincter dysfunction. Pudendal nerve terminal motor latency (PNTML) measures pudendal nerve function. With this procedure, a stimulating and recording electrode are utilized to measure the conduction of an impulse across the pudendal nerve.

Indications

Fecal incontinence and chronic constipation.

Complementary Procedures

Anorectal ultrasound, anorectal manometry, defecography, and flexible sigmoidoscopy.

Contraindications

Imperforate anus.

Relative Contraindications

A patient who is unable/unwilling to cooperate with the procedure.

Preparation of Patient

Some centers recommend a preparation of one or two Cleansing enemas prior to the procedure; others do not recommend any enemas as preparation for the procedure.

How the Procedure Is Performed

A physician places the electrode device over a gloved finger (a disposable model is available). This device has two stimulating electrodes at the tip of the gloved finger and two surface recording electrodes at the base of the finger. A grounding pad is applied to the patient's thigh. The finger is gently placed in the rectum with the tip of the finger pushing against the ischial spine. An electrical signal is given at the point of induction of contraction of the EAS, which may be felt by the examiner. The recording electrode then measures the latency separating the stimulating impulse and the contraction of the sphincter. This is termed the PNTML. Three readings are obtained at least three times on either side of the rectum. PNTML duration that is longer than 2.2 ± 0.2 ms is considered prolonged and is suggestive of pudendal nerve damage.

Typical Abnormal Findings

Prolonged PNTML is seen in patients with unexplained fecal incontinence. Unfortunately, it also appears to occur as a natural consequence of aging. Prolonged PNTML has been associated with pudendal nerve damage due to pelvic floor laxity and rectal prolapse. Recent studies have failed to demonstrate a relationship between descent of the perineum (a potential cause of obstructive constipation) and prolongation of PNTML.

Complications

None.

Additional Comments

This procedure is not recommended as a routine test in patients with chronic constipation or fecal incontinence due to a high rate of false-positive results in these patients.

Quantitative Stool Collection

Description of Procedure

In some patients with unexplained diarrhea, quantitative measurement of fecal volume, electrolytes, pH, and fat content over 24–72 h will assist in determining the cause of diarrhea. Stools may be spot tested for occult blood, white blood cells, parasites, pathogenic bacteria, and *C. difficile* toxin.

Indications

Chronic diarrhea with or without weight loss and nutritional deficiencies.

Complementary Procedures

Colonoscopy with biopsy of the mucosa, upper endoscopy with small intestinal biopsy, complete blood count, serum chemistry, thyroid-stimulating hormone levels, stool culture, D-xylose serum test, 24-h urine 5-hydroxyindole acetic acid (5-HIAA), small intestinal radiography, CT scan of the abdomen and pelvis, and serum hormone levels (vasoactive intestinal peptide, gastrin, somatostatin, and calcitonin).

Contraindications

None.

Relative Contraindications

Inability to collect stool specimens properly and to store over several days.

Preparation of Patient

For patients undergoing fecal fat testing, it is helpful to have a patient on a diet of 100 g fat/day. Patients should be given instructions regarding this diet. Patients should otherwise continue their usual activities.

How the Procedure Is Performed

All stools are collected over the designated time period using a special collection device that is placed over the toilet. Stools obtained during the collection period are stored in a sealed can containing a preservative. In between stool passages, the can with the collected stool is placed in a refrigerator. Patients keep a diary of all foods consumed during the collection period.

Typical Abnormal Findings

The collected stool is measured for volume and weight. Diarrhea is considered to be present if the volume is >200 mL/day or the weight is >200 g/day (see Table 2.2). The following electrolytes are commonly measured: sodium (Na), potassium (K), chloride (Cl), magnesium (Mg), and bicarbonate (HCO_3). The fecal osmotic gap is calculated with the following formula:

Fecal osmotic gap $= 290 - 2(Na + K)$.

A fecal osmotic gap of <50 suggests secretory diarrhea, while a fecal osmotic gap of >100 is characteristic of osmotic diarrhea. A fecal pH of <6 is suggestive of a malabsorptive disorder. In normal individuals, the total amount of fat in the stool should be <6% of the amount consumed. Thus, the presence of >6 g fat in the stool after consuming a 100 g fat diet suggests fat malabsorption. Very high fecal fat excretion (>20 g/day) is suggestive of pancreatic insufficiency. Elevated Mg in the stool can be found in laxative abusers. Additionally, the stool can be tested with a laxative screen using chromatography.

Table 2.2 Stool features in chronic diarrhea

Stools	Secretory	Osmotic	Inflammatory
Weight (g/day)	>1,000	500–1,000	<500
Osmolality	Normal	+	Normal
Osmotic gap	Normal	+	Normal
Na, CI	+	Normal	+
K; HCO_3	Low	Normal	Normal
Ph	High	Low	Normal

Complications

None.

Additional Comments

Although this procedure may be beneficial in diagnosing difficult cases of unexplained diarrhea, quantitative stool collection is cumbersome and is strongly disliked by patients and laboratory personnel.

Transanal Ultrasound

Description of Procedure

This is a transanal procedure involving placement of an ultrasonographic probe into the anus and rectum. The device rotates 360° for full evaluation of the IAS and EAS, as well as the rectum (compared to proctoscopy or sigmoidoscopy, which are used to view the mucosa only). Anorectal ultrasound has the advantage of evaluating all the tissue layers of the examined organs.

Indications

Evaluation of the anal sphincters in patients with fecal incontinence, staging of rectal cancers, evaluation of rectal lesions for evidence of invasion beyond the mucosa, and characterization of submucosal rectal lesions.

Complementary Procedures

Anorectal manometry, anorectal EMG, defecography, flexible sigmoidoscopy, colonoscopy, and barium enema.

Contraindications

Imperforate anus.

Relative Contraindications

Patient inability to cooperate with the procedure or severe anal stricture.

Preparation of Patient

The patient should receive two cleansing enemas 1–3 h before the procedure.

How the Procedure Is Performed

The patient is placed in a left lateral position. The ultrasonographic device is placed inside a hard plastic cover for evaluation of the anal canal, or inside a water-filled balloon for visualization of the rectum, and these are introduced into the anus. Ultrasound frequencies are transferred from the probe to a computer where they are reconstructed into a visual image. A resulting cross-sectional image of the anus and rectum is obtained. The IAS appears as a dark ring surrounded by a whitish ring representing the EAS. The mucosa, submucosa, lamina propria, muscularis mucosa, and serosa of the rectum can all be visualized as separate layers.

Typical Abnormal Findings

Transanal ultrasound can be used to evaluate the anatomy of the IAS and EAS. Sphincter injuries (due to obstetric damage, trauma, and prior surgeries) can be visualized (see Fig. 2.25). Thinning and degeneration of the anal sphincters may also be seen. The test may be used to evaluate patients who are being considered for sphincter repair for fecal incontinence. Transanal ultrasonography may be used to stage rectal carcinomas. Specifically, the test is accurate in determining whether the tumor is invading beyond the mucosa and the extent of this invasion. Enlargement of lymph nodes adjacent to the tumor may also be visualized. Therefore, this technique is useful in staging rectal tumors and for determining optimal medical and surgical management of the disease. Suspicious lymph nodes may also be sampled.

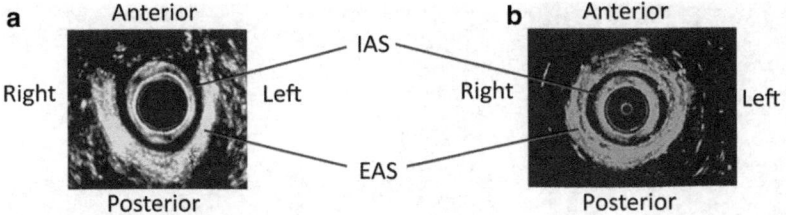

Fig. 2.25 (a) Anterior defect of IAS and EAS; (b) Normal IAS and EAS

Complications

Mild discomfort.

Additional Comments

This is an evolving technology. As with other forms of ultrasonography, the quality of information obtained from transanal ultrasonography is highly operator dependent.

CT Colonography

Procedure Overview

CT colonography (CTC), also known as virtual colonoscopy, is a minimally invasive, ultra-low radiation CT scan (typically done on a patient who underwent a saline cathartic preparation with oral contrast to tag residual fluid). It is performed to detect polyps and masses in the colon. Two- and three-dimensional images are reconstructed to search for polyps and to distinguish polyps from stool and other pitfalls of interpretation. Specialized training is critical in learning to recognize polyps and differentiating them from other structures (stool, folds, and other nonneoplastic findings). Colonic cleansing and gaseous distention (usually using carbon dioxide and a mechanical pump) is used to enhance the quality of the procedure (Fig. 2.26).

Indications

Screening or surveillance for colorectal polyps and masses, incomplete optical colonoscopy for any reason, searching for synchronous lesions in patients with known masses. Patients with relative contraindications for colonoscopy, for example,

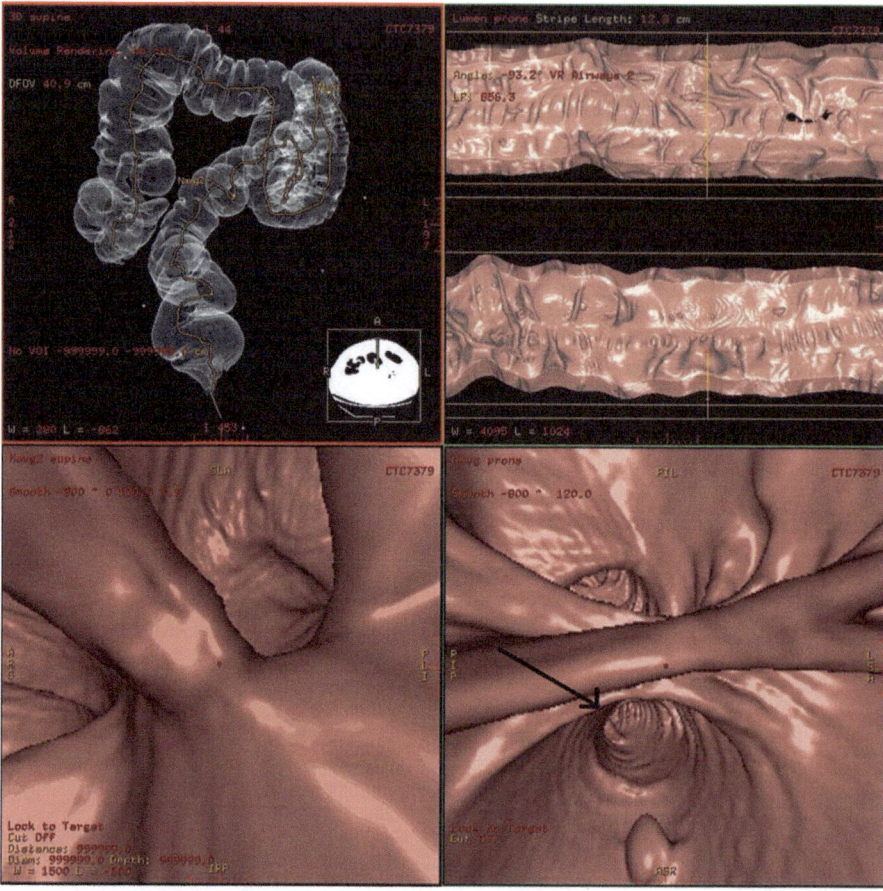

Fig. 2.26 Virtual colonoscopy. Example of a CTC display. Easy comparison of 2D and 3D images and of supine and prone images are critical to any CTC workstation. In this display: Upper left: 3D transparency overview of the colon shows the degree of tortuosity and can be used to mark polyp location to aid localization during follow-up endoscopy for patients with polyps. Lower: Supine and prone 3D endoluminal views. A polyp is seen on the prone view. Upper right: "Virtual dissection" view is one of several "novel display" options, which morph the colon to a flat surface for quick search for polyps. However, the polyps are therefore distorted (*arrow*)

on anticoagulation may prefer CTC. Uncommonly, to characterize indeterminate lesions found on optical colonoscopy, CTC can be done with intravenous contrast.

Complementary Procedures

Colonoscopy, flexible sigmoidoscopy, fecal occult blood testing, and fecal DNA testing.

Contraindications

Any reason to avoid raising intra-colonic pressure, for example, peritoneal signs, severe rectal bleeding, recent colon snare polypectomy, or electrocautery.

Relative Contraindications

Patients that would benefit from full colonoscopy including those with a high index of suspicion of colon cancer or polyps, known inflammatory bowel disease requiring surveillance or strong family history of colon cancer.

Preparation of Patient

Low-volume residue cathartic, for example, magnesium citrate, often with oral positive contrast tagging agents (low-density barium and or water soluble contrast). Polyethylene glycol-based colonic preparations can be used, although some deem this less desirable.

How the Procedure Is Performed

A thin catheter is placed in the rectum. The colon is insufflated with carbon dioxide using a pressure-sensitive mechanical pump for safety and comfort. Alternately, manual insufflation of room air can be used. The CT technologist must be trained to perform insufflation and recognize proper insufflation on the scout views. After insufflation, a scout view is performed to confirm adequate colonic distension. An ultra-low radiation dose CT is performed in a single short breathhold (16 slice scanner or better). This is repeated in the prone position. The technologist confirms that all segments of the colon are distended and that intraluminal fluid is properly tagged. If not, additional views can be obtained. The exam is interpreted on a dedicated 3D workstation by a trained radiologist.

Typical Abnormal Findings

Colon polyps and colon cancer. There are issues regarding the utility of this procedure as an alternative screening test compared to colonoscopy. Using multidetector scanners, meta-analysis suggests that the sensitivity of CTC for polyps greater than

10 mm is 82–100% and specificity of 90–98% for polyps greater or equal to 10 mm in diameter. Sensitivity and specificity are markedly decreased for smaller polyps. For example, it has been estimated that for polyps that are 6 mm or greater, CTC has a sensitivity of 86% and a specificity of 86%. The cost-effectiveness of reporting extracolonic findings is controversial, but significant actionable extracolonic findings are found in 5–9% of patients and up to 15% of medicare-aged patients undergoing CTC.

Complications

Pain, generally described as mild, from colonic distention or rare vasovagal reactions. Perforation is extremely rare. Pneumatosis intestinalis is also rare.

Additional Comments

Testing options for early detection of colorectal cancer and adenomatous polyps in asymptomatic adults 50 years of age and older have recently been published as a joint guideline from the American Cancer Society, the US Multi-Society Task Force on Colorectal Cancer, and the American College of Radiology. Options include fecal occult blood testing, flexible sigmoidoscopy, barium enema, CTC, and fecal DNA testing. Guidelines suggest that the sensitivity and specificity as well as ease of use of these tests vary, and the decision of which to use depends on a number of factors including availability, cost, and degree of invasive testing that patients wish to undergo for screening purposes. See American College of Radiology and American Gastroenterological Association white papers dealing with the subject and with training requirements. This chapter was written with the assistance of Dr Abraham Dachman, Department of Radiology, University of Chicago.

Chapter 3
Benign Anorectal Disorders

Eli D. Ehrenpreis

Anal Fissure

Definition

A tear, crack, or ulceration of the anal canal.

Epidemiology

An anal fissure can occur in any age group but is seen most commonly in young adults. They are found with equal frequency in males and females.

Patients at Risk

This condition may be brought on by the passage of a large, hard stool. It may occur more frequently in persons consuming low fiber, high fat diets. Anal fissures are also a feature of Crohn's disease, anorectal infections, leukemia, tuberculosis, and HIV infection.

E.D. Ehrenpreis, MD (✉)
Chief of Gastroenterology and Endoscopy, Highland Park Hospital,
NorthShore University Health System, Highland Park, IL 60035, USA

Clinical Associate Professor of Medicine, University of Chicago Medical Center,
Highland Park, IL 60035, USA
e-mail: ehrenpreis@gipharm.net

E.D. Ehrenpreis et al. (eds.), *Anal and Rectal Diseases: A Concise Manual*,
DOI 10.1007/978-1-4614-1102-4_3, © Springer Science+Business Media, LLC 2012

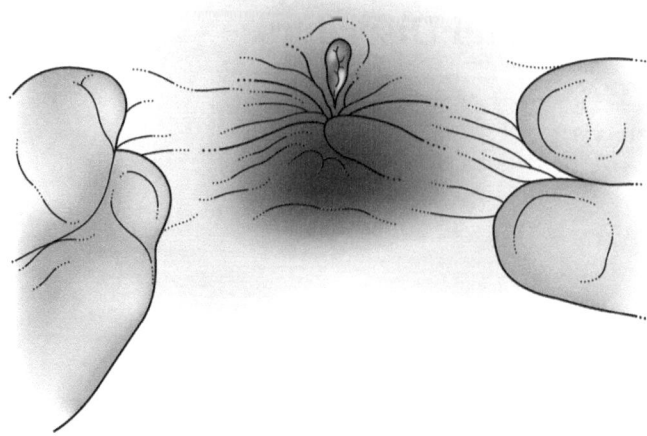

Fig. 3.1 Large anal fissure as seen in the typical posterior location (12 o'clock) on anal inspection

Pathophysiology

Anal fissures are most commonly seen in the posterior midline portion of the anal canal (see Fig. 3.1). This area may have decreased blood flow due to the configuration of the vasculature of the anus. Spasm of the internal anal sphincter may cause further reduction in blood flow to the posterior anal canal. This region of the anal canal has a higher risk of tearing because the arrangement of the anal muscles leads to less well-developed support of the anoderm in this region. Patients with a chronic anal fissure also appear to have increased resting and contracting pressures in the anus. Many also experience an anal sphincter spasm on defecation.

Symptoms

Pain and bleeding associated with defecation. The pain begins with defecation and persists after completion of the bowel movement. Bleeding is generally limited but may become severe and persistent.

Diagnosis

External examination is usually sufficient to make a diagnosis. Most fissures are seen posteriorly, however, 25% of fissures in women and 8% of fissures in men are anterior. Gentle separation of the buttocks to expose the perianal area may facilitate

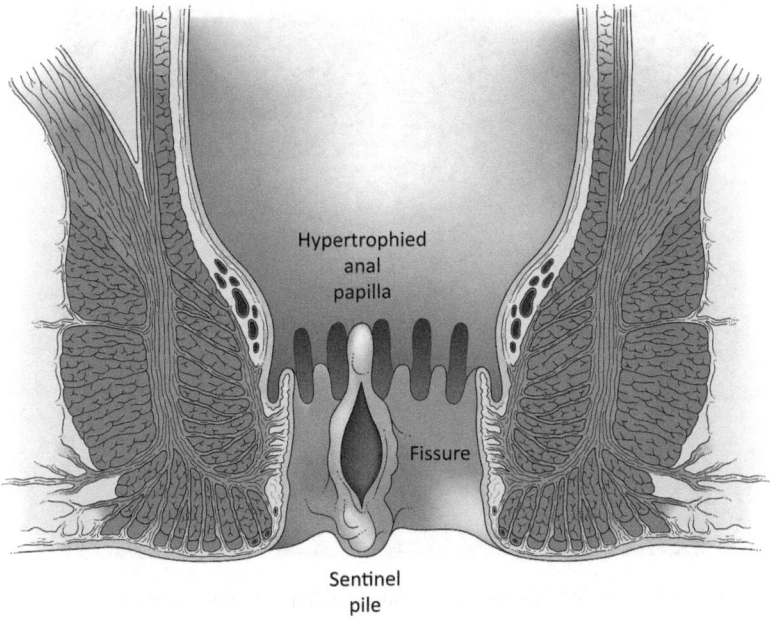

Fig. 3.2 Classic anatomic findings in chronic anal fissure including sentinel pile, fissure, and hypertrophied anal papilla

examination. Some patients may experience extreme physical discomfort on examination and may require anesthesia prior to full evaluation. Occasionally, anoscopy or flexible sigmoidoscopy is utilized (although these procedures may result in significant discomfort to the patient and may also require anesthesia).

Physical Findings

1. Sentinel pile (a small skin tag located outside of the anal canal near the fissure).
2. The fissure itself.
3. Hypertrophied anal papilla (originating at the dentate line) (see Figs. 3.2 and 3.3).

Treatment

Medical

First line: (45–87% healing rate). Stool softeners, fiber supplements such as psyllium (6–12 g/day) or bran (10–15 g/day), local anesthetic agents (such as lidocaine, benzocaine, or pramoxine), or warm sitz baths. Relaxation and avoidance of straining when going to the bathroom may be beneficial.

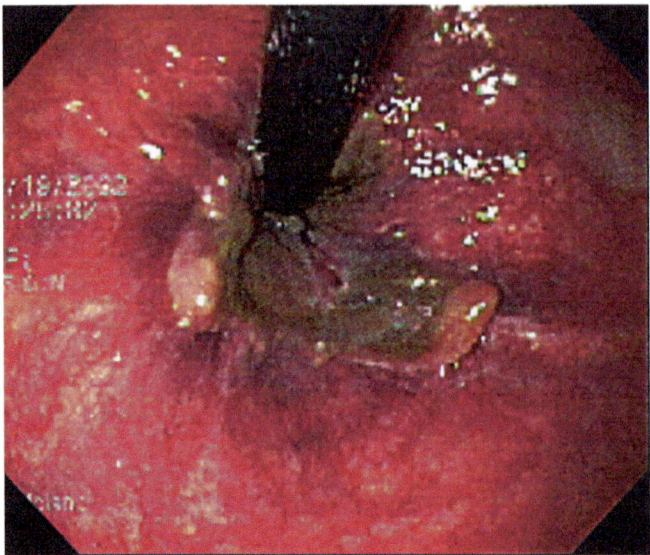

Fig. 3.3 Endoscopic view of a chronic anal fissure and hypertrophied anal papilla

Second line: (77–92% healing rate). Application of 0.2% topical nitroglycerin – this must be specially compounded by the pharmacist from standard 2% nitroglycerin mixed with petroleum jelly or another vehicle (such as glycerin). Approximately 1 g (enough to cover the tip of a gloved finger) should be applied 2–4 times/day to the anus. Patients should stay recumbent on their left side for 10–15 min after application due to the risk of hypotension from systemic nitroglycerin absorption. Topical calcium channel blockers such as 0.2% nifedipine and 2% diltiazem have shown beneficial effects similar to topical nitroglycerin. These are currently not available in the United States. Third line: (43–100% healing rate). Botulinum toxin (Botox 5–100 IU) may be injected into the internal anal sphincter using a small gauge needle and syringe. A method for endoscopic delivery of Botox injections into the internal anal sphincter has been developed by our practice. An upper endoscope is used to view the dentate line. Betadyne is used to cleanse the area and Botox is then injected lateral to the dentate line.

Surgical

Refractory patients require surgery. Surgical options include internal anal sphincterotomy with or without fissurectomy and manual dilatation of the anus, preferrably in the operating room. These procedures carry the risk of the development of fecal incontinence: reported postoperative risk of incontinence is between 0 and 38% with sphincterotomy and 8–12% with anal dilatation.

Clinical Pearls

An anal fissure becomes chronic when an acute tear progresses to the development of frank ulceration. The use of topical nitroglycerin and Botox therapy has greatly enhanced the medical management of chronic anal fissures.

Anal Stenosis

Definition

Narrowing of the anal canal.

Epidemiology

Anal stenosis can be congenital, but this is rare. Most commonly, anal stenosis is an acquired disorder associated with a variety of conditions. The most common cause of anal stenosis is prior hemorrhoidectomy.

Benign Causes

Prior hemorrhoidectomy, fissurectomy, anal sphincter repair, rectovaginal fistula repair, electrocautery for anal condyloma, prior anorectal radiation therapy, rectal foreign body insertion, trauma, chronic diarrhea, excessive laxative or mineral oil use, and Crohn's disease.

Malignant Causes

Anal or rectal carcinoma.

Pathophysiology

Excess anal skin utilization to close the wound after hemorrhoidectomy may cause stenosis. Carcinoma causes narrowing due to annular tumor growth. Scarring of the anus can occur secondary to Crohn's disease and as a complication of surgery.

Laxative use and diarrhea may cause narrowing of the anal canal from anal sphincter hypertrophy. Normally, anal sphincter muscle function is preserved and muscular hypertrophy prevented by the presence of solid fecal boluses that intermittently cause dilatation and relaxation of the anal sphincter.

Symptoms

Narrowing of the stool, passage of small stools, incomplete evacuation, painful defecation, and hematochezia (passage of red blood from the rectum) are symptoms of anal stenosis.

Diagnosis

Diagnosis is via digital rectal examination. Difficulty of passage of the finger into the rectum occurs because of decreased anal diameter. Additional tests may include anoscopy, flexible sigmoidoscopy, colonoscopy, barium enema, or pelvic imaging, e.g., a computed tomography (CT) scan. Biopsies are obtained to rule out malignancy. Anorectal ultrasound may improve visualization of the anal canal to rule out malignancy. Examination under anesthesia may be required.

Treatment

Medical

Bulking agents, stool softeners, and periodic dilatation using a digital method or flexible dilators of increasing diameter.

Surgical

In cases of scarring, removal of the scar in combination with sphincterotomy. Anoplasty (the use of perianal skin to cover an area of the anal canal) is used for moderate – severe cases.

Clinical Pearls

In appropriately selected candidates, surgery appears to be the treatment of choice since stool bulking and anal dilatation are primarily temporizing and do not correct the narrowing of the anal canal.

Anorectal Abscess

Definition

An infection that begins in the anal glands and extends into spaces around the anus and rectum.

Epidemiology

Anorectal abscesses are most common in adults between the ages of 20 and 40 years. Twice as many males have this condition as females. Anorectal abscesses may occur in association with a variety of medical illnesses.

Patients at Risk

Anorectal abscesses are more common in patients with a variety of chronic medical conditions compared to the general population. Patients at risk include those with Crohn's disease, diabetes, heart disease, lymphoma, leukemia, anal and rectal cancer, radiation proctopathy, hidradenitis suppurativa, and infections of the perianal region. Anorectal abscesses can be caused by a variety of infections including *Chlamydia* infection, actinomycosis, and tuberculosis.

Pathophysiology

By definition, an anorectal abscess is a collection of pus in the perianal or perirectal region (see Fig. 3.4). The process is most likely initiated by obstruction of the anal glands followed by infections with the above-mentioned organisms or colonic bacteria. Infections may then expand into a variety of spaces within the anorectal region. The four most important locations where pus may accumulate are the perianal, ischiorectal, intersphincteric, and supralevator spaces (see Fig. 3.5).

Symptoms

The most common symptoms are pain and swelling in the anorectal region. Anal discharge and anorectal bleeding may be present.

Fig. 3.4 Perianal abscess
with a small perianal wart
opposite

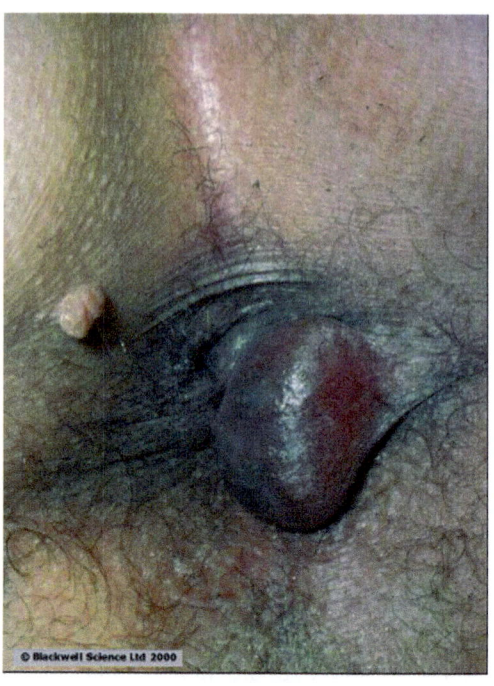

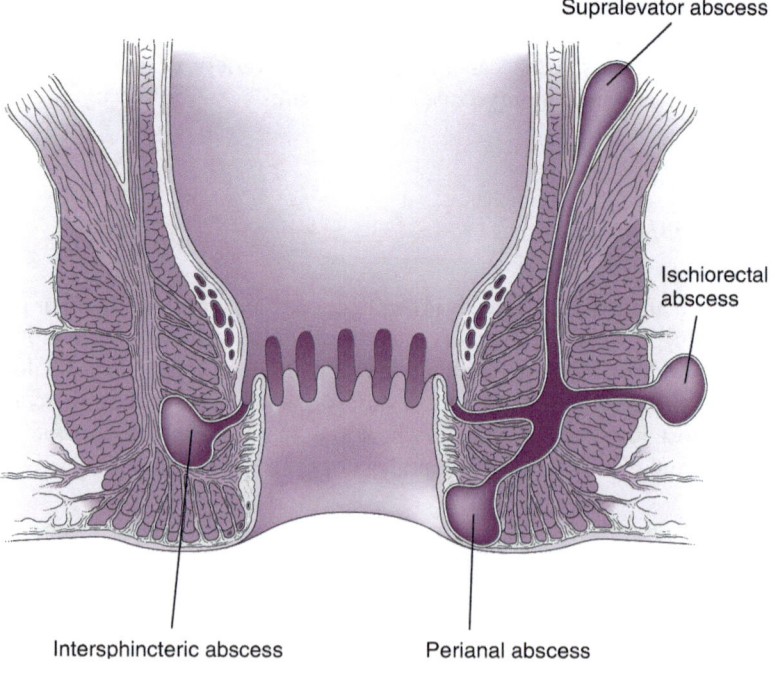

Fig. 3.5 Classification of anorectal abscesses

Diagnosis

The diagnosis is made by taking appropriate history and physical examination. Examination reveals a swollen, tender, erythematous, and warm enlargement in the perianal region. Some drainage may be present and a pin-like opening may be revealed. Anesthesia may be required to complete the examination, including a digital rectal evaluation.

Treatment

All anorectal abscesses require drainage (see Chap. 9). This may be performed in the operating room or at the bedside depending on the location and severity of the abscess. Excision of a fistula associated with the abscess may be required at a later stage.

Culturing of the material collected after drainage is suggested for individuals who are immunocompromised. Subsequent treatment with Sitz™ baths, stool softeners, a high-fiber diet, laxatives, and local bandaging may be required. Treatment of the underlying disease is also beneficial.

Clinical Pearls

In routine cases of anorectal abscesses, preoperative and postdrainage antibiotics are only recommended in immunocompromised patients and individuals with valvular heart disease.

Constipation

This is a symptom most objectively defined as fewer than three spontaneous bowel movements per week. Other definitions include decreased stool bulk, change in stool caliber (diameter), and straining with stool passage.

Epidemiology

Large national surveys in the United States including the National Health Interview Survey (NHIS) and the National Health and Nutrition Examination Survey (NHANES) suggest that between 2 and 13% of the population of the United States report the symptom of constipation to their physician each year. According to the NHANES, 3.2% of males and 9.1% of females have fewer than three bowel movements per week. Studies in the United Kingdom suggest that the prevalence of constipation is between 8 and 13%.

Patients at Risk

Constipation becomes more common with advancing age: prevalence in developed countries increases to 25% in the elderly. The rate of physician visits for the complaint of constipation increases from 1.3% for younger patients to 4.1% annually for persons over the age of 65 years. Symptoms of constipation are approximately 3 times more common in women than in men. Constipation appears to be more common in individuals of lower socioeconomic status and occurs less frequently in the white population.

Pathophysiology

Causes of constipation may be divided into several categories, these are outlined below.

Slow Colonic Transit

Decreased motility resulting from neuromuscular dysfunction. Causes include medications (anticholinergics, calcium channel blockers, opioids [see Fig. 3.6]), Chagas' disease, Hirschsprung's disease, and endocrinopathies such as diabetes and hypothyroidism. Idiopathic colonic inertia is a syndrome seen predominantly in young women and may be due to a neuromyopathy.

Obstructive Defecation (Pelvic Floor Disorders)

These may be due to anorectal muscle spasm (nonrelaxing puborectalis syndrome, anismus), prolapses (rectal prolapse, anorectal intussusception), rectoceles (see Figs. 3.7 and 3.8), or pelvic laxity. These disorders are most commonly seen in women.

Mechanical Obstruction

Strictures (carcinoma, radiation-induced, Crohn's disease, diverticular, ischemic).

Psychogenic

Patients may feel compelled to have daily bowel movements (due to an abnormal concern about regularity).

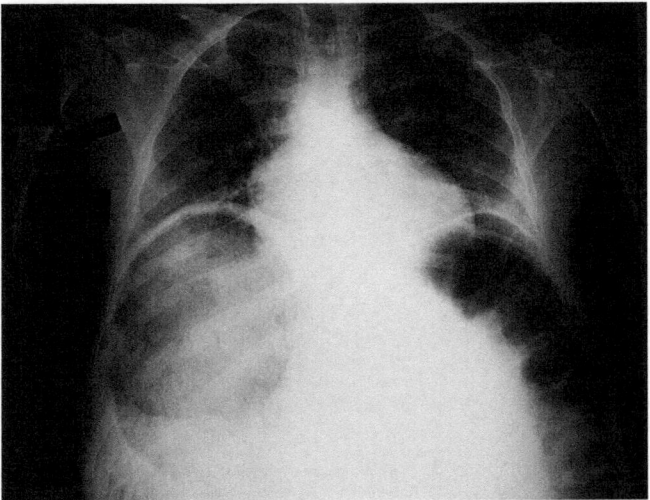

Fig. 3.6 Abdominal plain radiograph demonstrates dilated left and right colon in a patient on chronic opiod therapy

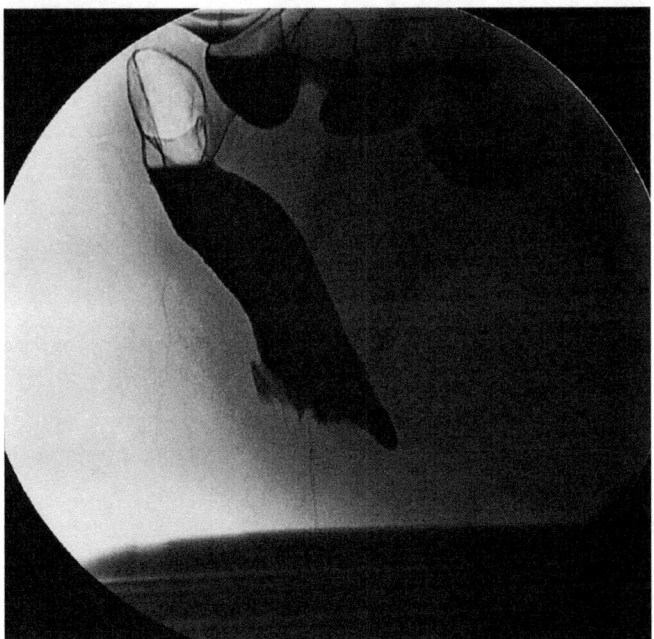

Fig. 3.7 Rectocele demonstrated on dynamic protography

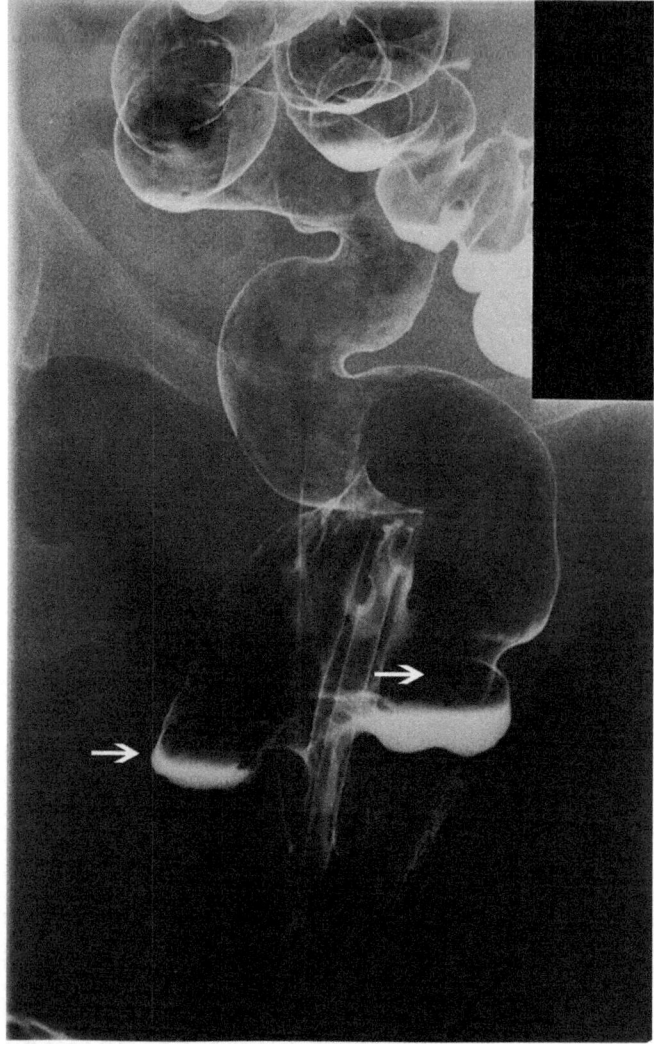

Fig. 3.8 Lateral rectoceles (*arrows*) demonstrated on dynamic proctography. The Patient complained of difficulty with evacuation

Symptoms

When daily bowel movements do not occur, patients may complain of decreased stool frequency, decreased stool bulk, narrow stools, and/or straining with stool passage.

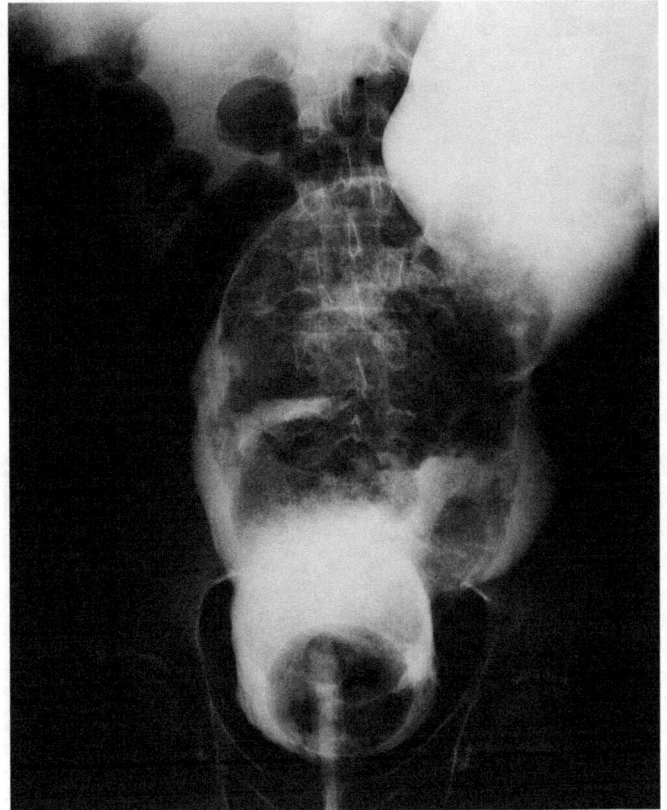

Fig. 3.9   Megarectum demonstrated on barium enema in a patient with chronic constipation

Diagnosis

Laboratory

Complete blood count, thyroid stimulating hormone, and serum electrolytes.

Anatomic

Colonoscopy, barium enema (see Fig. 3.9), flexible sigmoidoscopy, or anoscopy.

Physiologic (Obstructive Defecation)

Dynamic proctography, anorectal manometry, nerve conduction velocity, electromyography (EMG), and sitz marker study (see Figs. 3.10–3.12).

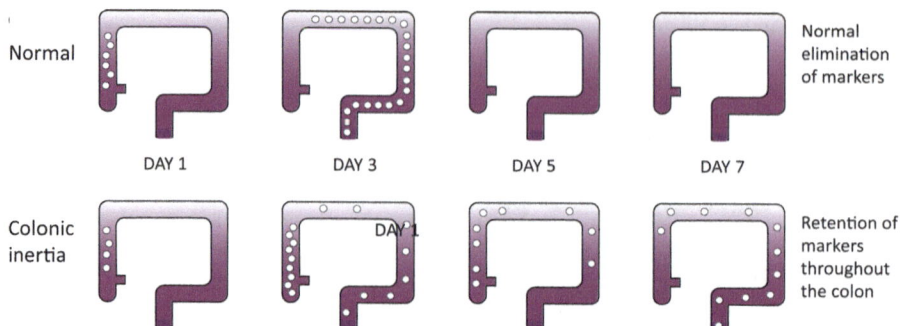

Fig. 3.10 Movement of Sitz™ markers in the colon in normal subjects and patients with colonic inertia. Patients with colonic inertia have accumulation of markers throughout the colon on day 5 after ingestion

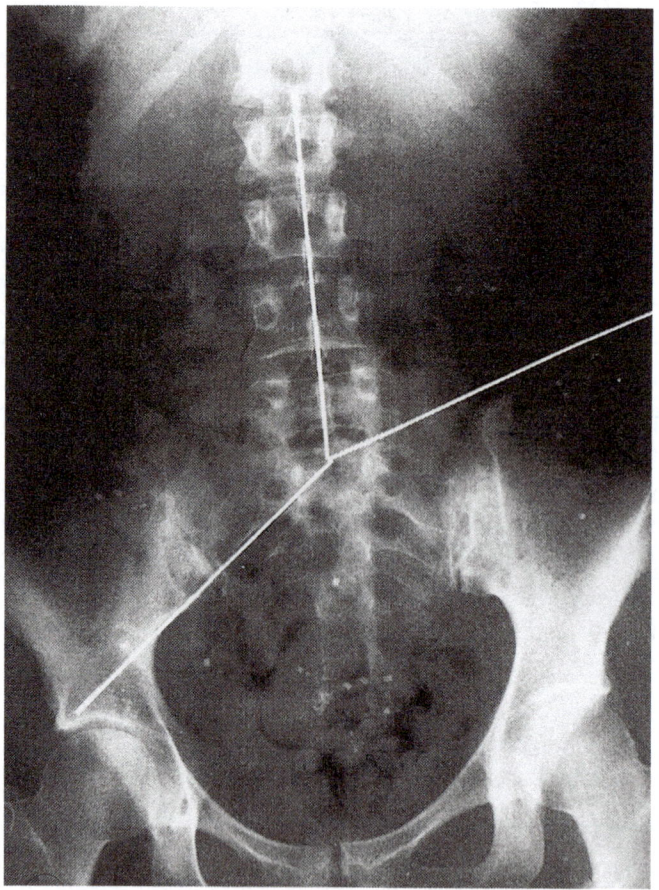

Fig. 3.11 Sitz™ marker study on day 5 in a constipated patient demonstrates markers throughout the colon. Lines separate the right, middle, and left colon. Marker distribution patterns vary depending on the cause of constipation

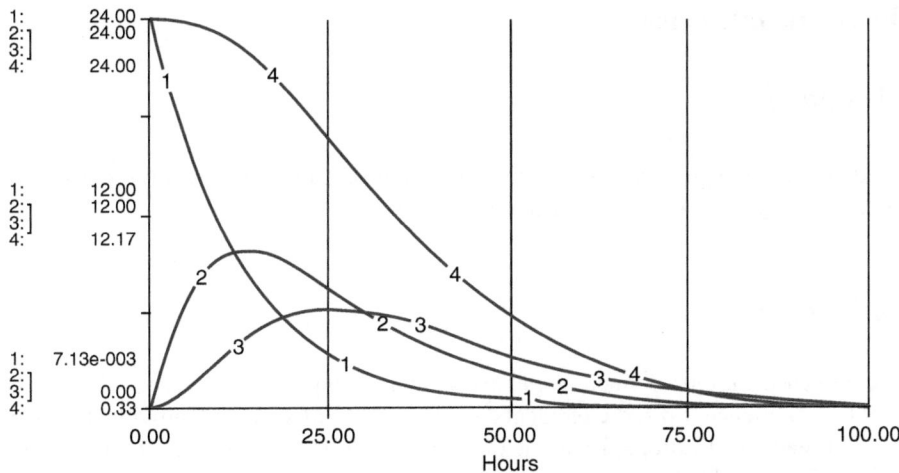

Fig. 3.12 Simulation of segmental colonic transit of Sitz™ markers based on data from 20 normal volunteers (1: right colon; 2: left colon; 3: rectosigmoid colon; 4: colon) using a dynamic computer model

Other

Full thickness rectal biopsy (in patients with suspected Hirschsprung's disease).

Treatment

Fiber therapy, laxatives, stool softeners, lactulose and sorbitol, polyethylene glycol plus electrolytes, biofeedback therapy, botulinum toxin (Botox) injections, surgical repair of rectocele (see Chap. 10), subtotal colectomy and ileorectal anastomosis for colonic inertia, and lateral internal anal sphincterotomy.

Clinical Pearls

Taking a careful history will assist in differentiating the various causes of constipation. In general, an anatomic evaluation of the large intestine with a barium enema or colonoscopy should be included in the evaluation to screen for colon polyps, colonic strictures, and malignancies.

Fecal Incontinence

Definition

Inadvertent passage of rectal contents, including soiling of underclothing or involuntary passage of gas, mucus, or liquid/solid stool.

Epidemiology

Incontinence may be defined as gas incontinence, liquid incontinence, or formed stool incontinence. Episodic incidents occur in 2–7% of surveyed individuals in the United States and Europe. Frank incontinence of solid stool is rarer and is seen in 0.7% of surveyed individuals in the United States and Europe. Fecal incontinence is most common in older women, and is the second most common cause of nursing home placement in the elderly. About 25% of patients with diarrhea-predominant irritable bowel syndrome have episodes of fecal incontinence. Patients often avoid reporting the symptom of fecal incontinence.

Patients at Risk

The elderly, patients with neurologic disease or injury, prior anorectal surgery, prior anorectal obstetric trauma, receptive traumatic anal intercourse, other anorectal trauma, colitis, chronic diarrhea, fecal impaction, or congenital anomalies.

Pathophysiology

Incontinence occurs when normal anorectal function is disrupted. Damage to the anal sphincter, diseases of sensory and motor neurons of the pelvis, altered sensorium, and spinal cord injury may all result in leakage of stool due to inadequate sensation of the presence of stool in the rectum. Fecal soiling may occur in the elderly from constipation and overflow incontinence.

Symptoms

Classification by the type of incontinence and severity is important for determining the treatment regimen. Classification should be made on the basis of the factors shown in Table 3.1.

Table 3.1 Factors determining severity of incontinence type

Contents	Gas, liquid, or solid stool
Frequency	Rare, occasional, usual, or constant
Wearing of a pad	Rare, occasional, usual, or constant
Effects on lifestyle	Mild, moderate, or severe

Diagnosis

Digital rectal examination to identify resting tone and sphincter deformities; anorectal manometry to measure resting and squeeze pressures; anorectal ultrasound to visualize the sphincter for injury or other deformities; EMG and pudendal nerve terminal motor latency (PNTML) for detecting neuromuscular damage.

Treatment

Medical

- Antidiarrheal agents including loperamide, diphenoxylate, codeine, and other opiates
- Anticholinergic agents including hyoscyamine, dicyclomine, atropine, and clindium
- Fiber supplements, particularly calcium polycarbophyl
- Other constipating agents including cholestyramine
- Performance of Kegel exercises
- Biofeedback therapy

Procedural

A system called Secca® (Mederi Therapeutics Inc) (see Fig. 3.13) utilizes the delivery of radiofrequency waves into the anal sphincter. The technique results in remodeling of sphincter muscles and appears to improve symptoms (see Chap. 11).

Surgical

Surgical options include, but are not limited to overlapping sphincter muscle repair, gracilis muscle transposition with and without neuromuscular stimulation, artificial bowel sphincter, and colostomy (see Chap. 11).

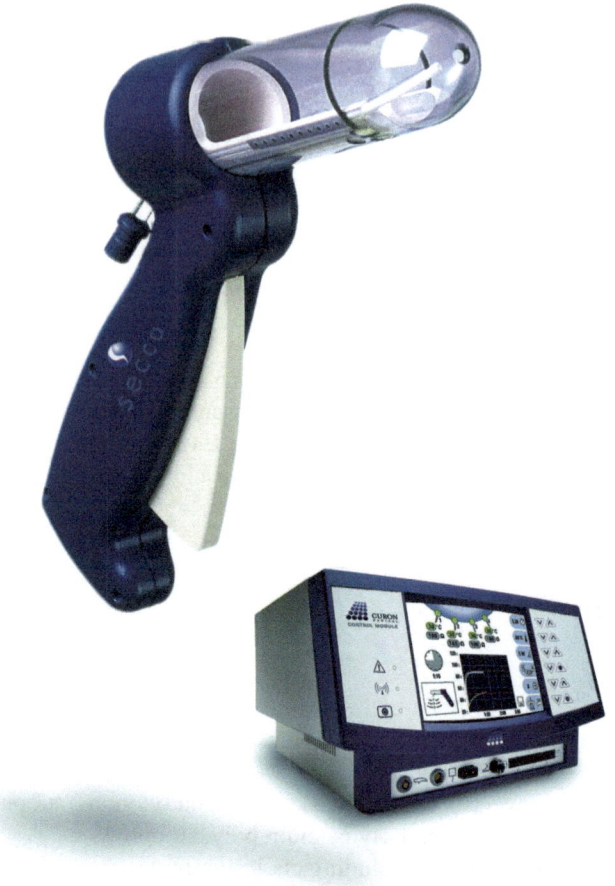

Fig. 3.13 The Secca System for fecal incontinence

Clinical Pearls

Daily laxatives combined with enema therapy once per week have been shown to effectively reduce incontinence episodes in elderly patients with overflow incontinence.

Hemorrhoids

Definition

Dilation of anal venous structures.

Fig. 3.14 Internal
hemorrhoid as seen
on anoscopy

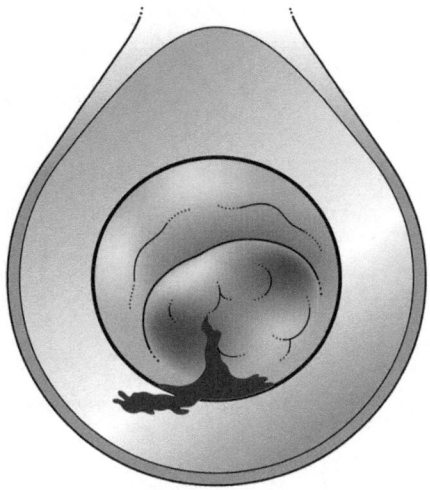

Epidemiology

Hemorrhoids occur in up to 50% of the adult population.

Anatomy

Internal

Internal hemorrhoids are dilatations of the venous structures in the internal hemorrhoidal plexus (see Figs. 3.14, 3.15). The veins are lined with rectal mucosa (transitional and columnar epithelium), which contains limited pain fibers. Internal hemorrhoids
originate from above the dentate line (see Anal and Rectal Anatomy Chapt. 1).

External

External hemorrhoids arise from the inferior venous plexus. They are lined with
perianal squamous endothelium and contains a large number of pain fibers. External
hemorrhoids originate from below the dentate line.

Patients at Risk

The elderly and those with straining secondary to chronic constipation, pregnancy,
pelvic malignancy, chronic obstructive pulmonary disease with chronic cough,
chronic diarrhea, and a variety of diseases or syndromes that increase the venous
pressure within the pelvis.

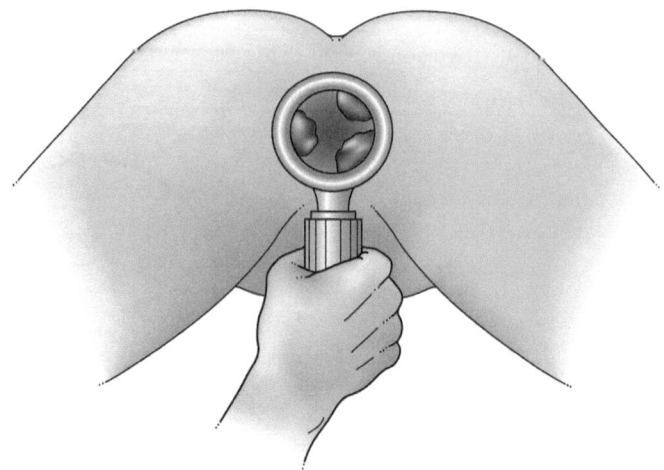

Fig. 3.15 The main locations of internal hemorrhoids: right, anterior, right posterior, and left lateral

Pathophysiology

Hemorrhoids are made up of blood vessels, connective tissue, and lining tissue (rectal or anal mucosa). Aging and straining reduce the ability of the connective tissue to provide adequate support for hemorrhoids resulting in their dilatation and decreased venous return. Inflammation of overlying mucosa may contribute to symptomatology.

Complications

Internal Hemorrhoids

Bleeding.

First-degree prolapse: internal hemorrhoids move into the anal canal.
Second-degree prolapse: prolapse of hemorrhoids outside the anal canal with straining, which resolves spontaneously.
Third-degree prolapse: hemorrhoids protrude outside of the anal canal and require replacement by digital maneuvers.
Fourth-degree prolapse: hemorrhoids protrude outside the anal canal and cannot be manually reduced.

External Hemorrhoids

Thrombosis: by definition, this occurs when a clot is present in an external hemorrhoid (see Fig. 3.16). Secondary inflammation, bleeding, and ulceration may follow.

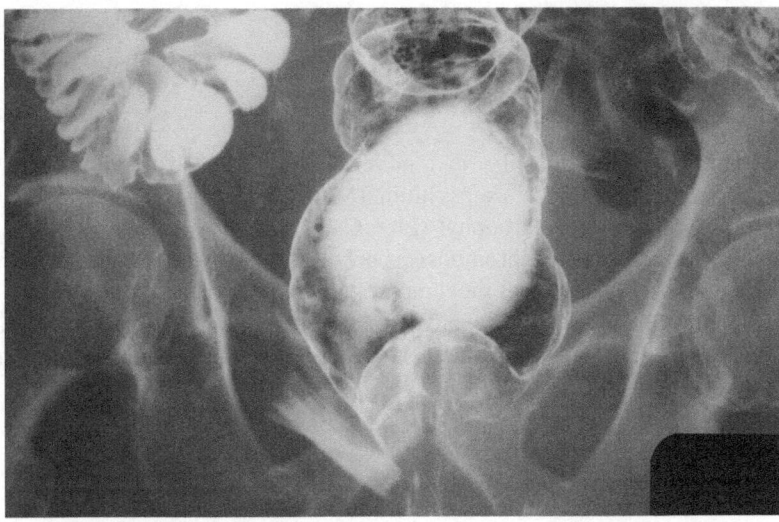

Fig. 3.16 Thrombosed hemorrhoid. Rare barium study demonstrates filling defect

Symptoms

Internal Hemorrhoids

Sensation of prolapse, mild discomfort, soiling, passage of small quantities of bright red blood. Severe pain associated with prolapse may suggest strangulation of prolapsed internal hemorrhoids. This is a serious, potentially life-threatening condition.

External Hemorrhoids

Pain (primarily with thrombosis). Presence of external skin tag and pruritus ani.

Diagnosis

Perianal examination is used initially. Prolapse may be demonstrated by having the patient perform a straining maneuver. Gentle palpation is used to diagnose thrombosis of external hemorrhoids. Anoscopy or sigmoidoscopy is required to diagnose internal hemorrhoids that are not prolapsed.

Treatment

General

Internal hemorrhoids: a high-fiber diet, increased fluids, and avoidance of straining. Add fiber supplements such as psyllium (Metamucil, Konsyl), methylcellulose (Citrucel), or calcium polycarbophyl (FiberCon). Sitz™ baths relieve discomfort. External hemorrhoids: when thrombosis is present, sitz baths are recommended 3–4 times/day and after each bowel movement. A high-fiber diet, stool softeners, fiber supplementation as above, and laxatives may be beneficial. Patients should avoid straining. Topical local anesthetic creams (such as lidocaine, benzocaine, or pramoxine) should be applied 2–4 times/day.

Nonsurgical, Procedural

These treatments are utilized for internal hemorrhoids only. They are most effective for first- and second-degree prolapsed hemorrhoids. Rubber band ligation: this is an outpatient procedure performed after placement of an anoscope. A specialized device grabs the hemorrhoid and places a rubber band tightly around it (see Fig. 3.17). Complications associated with this technique include pain (sometimes resulting in the need to remove the rubber band), bleeding from early dislodgment of the rubber bands, infection, and perirectal abscess. Severe necrotizing infection from gas-forming organisms is a very rare reported complication.

Injection: this is a form of sclerotherapy using a sclerosing agent. The chemical is injected near the hemorrhoids causing an inflammatory reaction and a clot within the hemorrhoid. Complications associated with this technique include infection, ulceration, and pain.

Photocoagulation: this method uses infrared light to produce venous thrombosis and scarring. This technique is easily performed as an outpatient procedure without sedation and is well tolerated. Complications associated with this technique include pain and ulceration.

Other methods: cryosurgery, electrocoagulation, and saline injections.

Surgical

Internal hemorrhoids: most colorectal surgeons agree that third- and fourth-degree hemorrhoids require hemorrhoidectomy. Stapled hemorrhoidectomy has been recently introduced and involves the use of circular staples applied above (proximal to) the dentate line. Early studies have shown that this technique is associated with less postoperative pain than conventional hemorrhoidectomy.

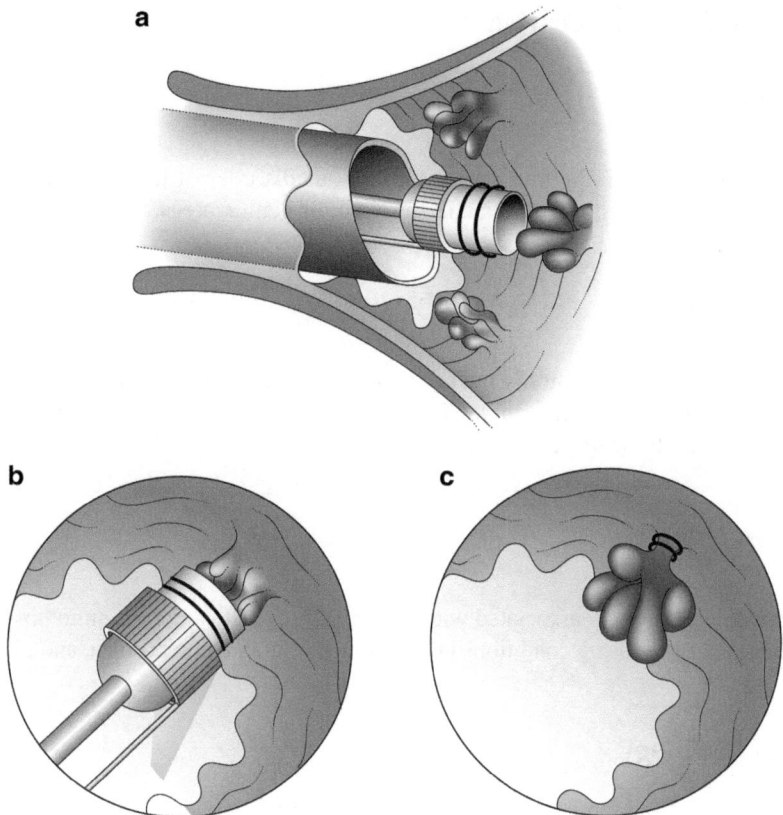

Fig. 3.17 Technique for rubber band ligation of internal hemorrhoids. (**a**) The aspirator-ligator is inserted through an anoscope. (**b**) Suction is applied, pulling the mucosa and venous plexus into the suction cup. (**c**) The ligator is fired and two rubber bands are applied. Only one or two areas are banded in a single session

External hemorrhoids: surgery is utilized in patients who have pain that is severe and/or lasts >48 h. Treatment involves either removal of the thrombosis or excision of the hemorrhoid. Thrombectomy alone cannot be performed after approximately 48 h (see Chap. 12).

Clinical Pearls

It is important to differentiate hemorrhoids from anorectal varices, which occur in patients with preexisting portal hypertension. Like external hemorrhoids, anorectal varices begin below the dentate line then expand into the rectum. Bleeding anorectal varices are most often treated with nonsurgical procedures such as rubber band ligation, as described for internal hemorrhoids.

Hidradenitis Suppurativa

Definition

An acute or chronic inflammatory and infectious disorder of the apocrine (sweat) glands. It often occurs in the perianal, inguinal, or genital areas.

Epidemiology

This condition most commonly occurs in younger individuals, between the ages of 16–45 years. It is more common in women. However, perineal involvement requiring surgery appears to be more common in men.

Patients at Risk

This condition is closely associated with Crohn's disease. It is more common in blacks than whites. Predisposing conditions include diabetes mellitus, seborrhea, and obesity.

Pathophysiology

The process is initiated when an apocrine duct becomes obstructed by keratinous secretions. This results in expansion of the sweat gland and secondary infection from skin flora and colonic bacteria. Rupture of the gland leads to involvement of adjacent areas and spreading of the infection (see Fig. 3.18). The most common site of involvement is the axilla. The next most commonly involved sites are the perianal and genital regions. Poor skin hygiene and a prior history of acne may predispose to the development of the condition.

Symptoms

Patients develop pruritus, pain, and leakage from the affected area.

Diagnosis

Physical examination reveals multiple lesions at affected sites. Lesions are erythematous and tender to palpation. A purulent discharge may be present. Extensive sinus formation with palpable abscesses and a honeycomb-like distribution of the lesions may be seen in the region of the anus, genitalia, gluteus, and thighs.

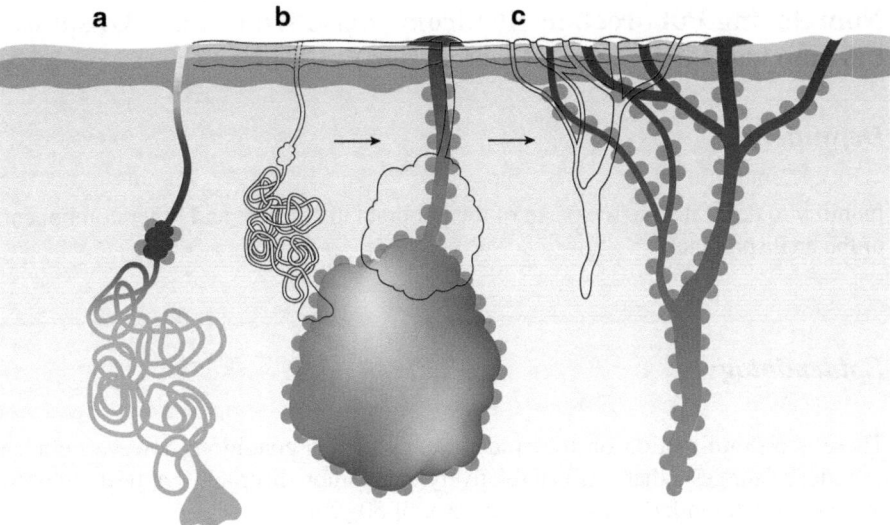

Fig. 3.18 Hidradenitis suppurative. (**a**) The first event is blockage of an apocrine duct by a keratinous plug. (**b**) Bacteria trapped beneath the plug multiply to form an abscess, with rupture into
adjacent tissue. (**c**) Subsequently, recurrent abscesses, draining sinuses, and indurated scarred skin
and subcutaneous tissues occur

Treatment

Cleansing of affected areas may be beneficial. Discontinuation of oral contraceptive
therapy has been effective in some patients. Antibiotic therapy with coverage for
skin and colon flora may be effective in early disease. Suitable antibiotics include
tetracycline, erythromycin, Augmentin (amoxicillin/clavulanate potassium), and
penicillin. Oral isotretinoin has been effective in a small number of patients. Topical
clindamycin has also been helpful, as have topical and intralesional injections
with steroids. Surgical management for nonresponsive patients involves excision
of the sinuses, sometimes with application of a graft to the surgical wound (see
Chap. 13).

Clinical Pearls

Hidradenitis suppurativa may be confused with infections of the perianal region,
sebaceous cysts, and perianal Crohn's disease.

Nonrelaxing Puborectalis Syndrome (Also Known as: Anismus, Paradoxical Puborectalis Contraction)

Definition

Inability to defecate due to spasm of the puborectalis muscle and other components of the anal sphincter.

Epidemiology

There is no information on the epidemiology of this condition; however, clinical experience suggests that this is a relatively uncommon disorder. It appears to occur more frequently in individuals over the age of 50 years.

Patients at Risk

This condition may be associated with anxiety and obsession regarding bowel habits. Patients with a history of sexual abuse appear to be at higher risk for developing the condition, however, the reason for this is unknown.

Pathophysiology

The puborectalis muscle attaches to the pubic bone and envelops the distal rectum in a sling-like fashion, forming the anorectal angle. It is a skeletal muscle, which is normally in a contracted state at rest. The anorectal angle assists with maintaining continence. The puborectalis muscle relaxes at the time of defecation, thus increasing the anorectal angle, allowing stool to move distally for evacuation. People with this condition are unable to relax the puborectalis muscle and external anal sphincter, thus developing a form of pelvic floor obstruction and constipation.

Symptoms

Difficulty with evacuation, straining, and incomplete evacuation are the most common symptoms. The passage of multiple small stools with marked straining may also suggest this diagnosis.

Diagnosis

Physical examination with digital rectal examination may reveal the diagnosis. Patients are asked to push to assist evacuation of the finger within the rectum. Lack of relaxation of the sphincter with this maneuver may suggest the presence of non-relaxing puborectalis syndrome. However, a number of authors have cautioned that this physical finding is only suggestive of the diagnosis. Anorectal manometry, dynamic proctography, and anorectal EMG are the most useful diagnostic tests for this condition. Some authors have suggested that dynamic proctography and ano-rectal manometry should both be performed if the nonrelaxing puborectalis syn-drome is suspected, since each test performed individually lacks sensitivity and specificity.

Treatment

Patient education may be of some benefit. Fiber supplementation is beneficial, and injection of 6–100 IU of botulinum toxin (Botox) into the puborectalis mus-cle or internal anal sphincter region has recently been shown to be successful in a small number of patients. Biofeedback therapy has proven to be beneficial in up to 90% of patients. Surgical management may be an option for some patients; however, only a limited number of surgical studies have been performed. For example, a small group of patients appears to have benefited from lateral divi-sion of the puborectalis muscle. A small number of patients also appear to have benefited from dilatation of the anal sphincter with dilators of increasing diameter.

Clinical Pearls

Sphincter nonrelaxation on anorectal manometry and defecography may occur in patients who are excessively nervous when undergoing these procedures. Our group has demonstrated a beneficial effect of Botox injection into the internal anal sphincter via an endoscopic route for patients with spasmic anorectal disorders.

Nonrelaxing puborectalis syndrome is not associated with anorectal pain. It is important to consider the diagnosis of levator ani syndrome in patients com-plaining of pain and difficulty with evacuation. Patients with levator ani syn-drome will have marked tenderness of the anal sphincter on digital rectal examination.

Perianal Crohn's Disease

Definition

The development of a variety of pathologic conditions of the perianal region such as fistulas, abscesses, and strictures caused by inflammation from Crohn's disease (see Fig. 3.19).

Epidemiology

Perianal symptoms occur in more than 40% of patients with Crohn's disease. Perianal pathology includes the development of fistulas, anal fissures, and abscesses. Perianal fistulas are seen in 28% of patients with Crohn's disease. Enlarged, thickened anal skin tags are frequently present and form de novo as a direct effect of local inflammation (see Fig. 3.20).

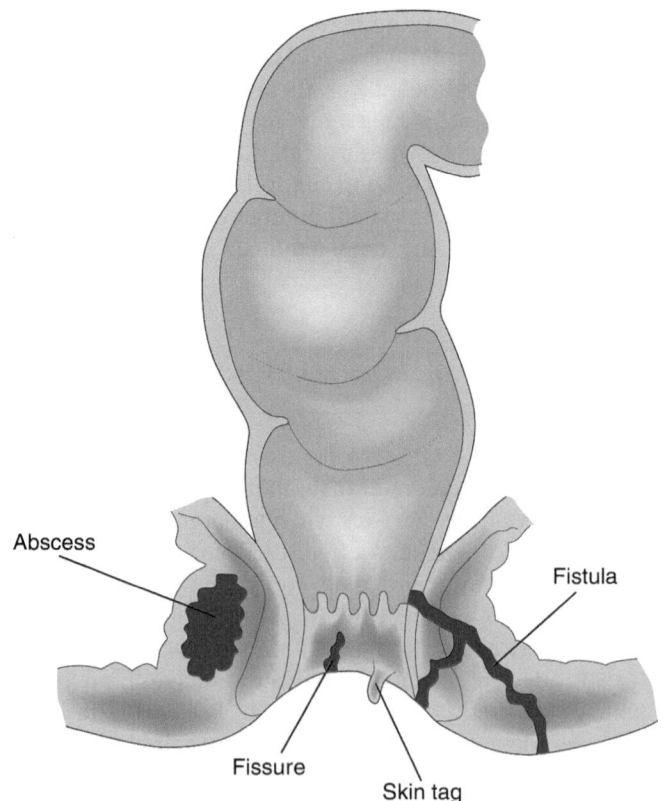

Fig. 3.19 Anorectal disorders seen in patients with Crohn's disease

Patients at Risk

Perianal involvement is more common in patients with rectal Crohn's disease (92%) and colonic Crohn's disease (52%) than in those with small intestinal Crohn's disease (14%). Patients with Crohn's proctitis are at particular risk for perianal fistulas. A symptomatic perianal fistula is the initial clinical presentation in about 5% of patients with Crohn's disease.

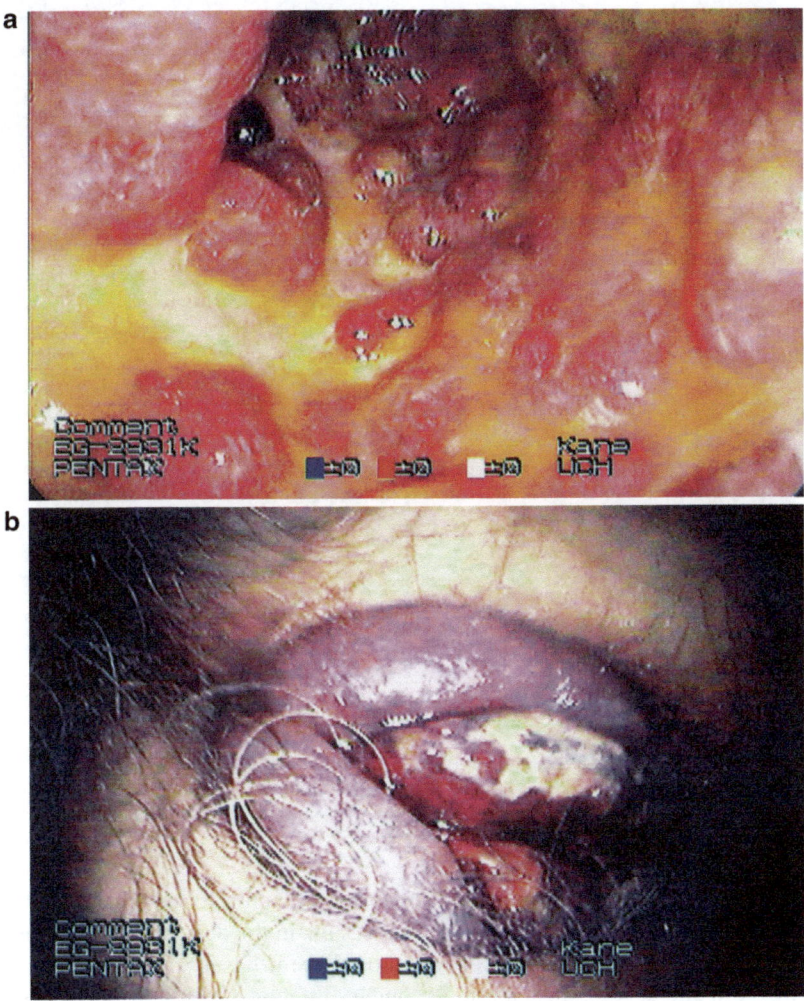

Fig. 3.20 Perianal Crohn's disease with large skin tags, perianal inflammation, proctitis, and thrombosed hemorrhoids (photo courtesy of Dr. Sunanda V. Kane)

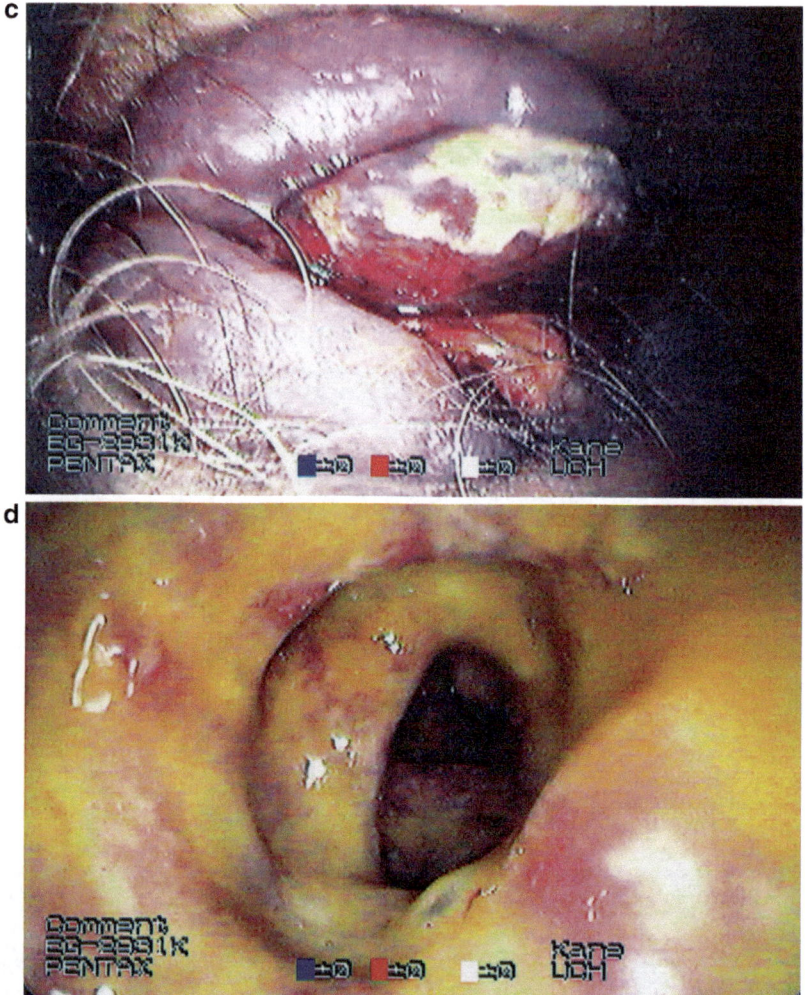

Fig. 3.20 (continued)

Pathophysiology

Transmural, chronic inflammation of the gut wall extends to local tissues. Secretion of proteases and other destructive enzymes results in the development of sinus cavities. Anal gland inflammation extends into adjacent tissues, which results in anal fistulization and abscess formation. Secondary infection within these spaces occurs due to exposure to colonic bacteria. Complex fistulas are a distinguishing feature of perianal Crohn's disease.

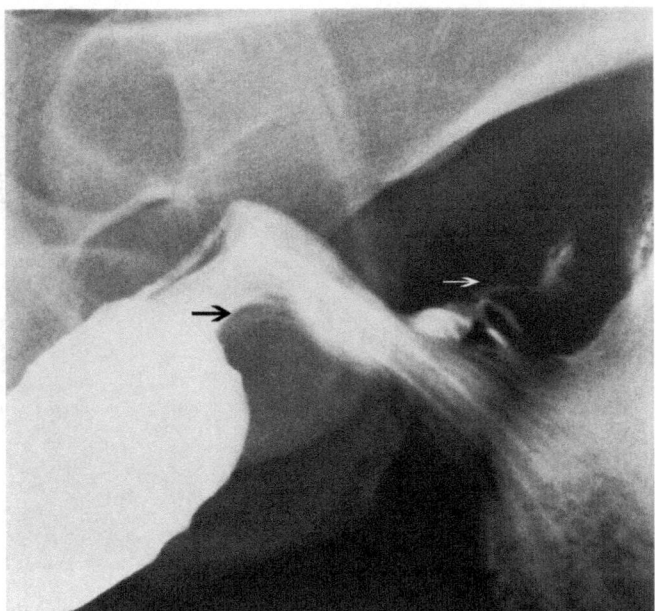

Fig. 3.21 Lateral view of an anovaginal fistula (*small arrow*) in a patient with Crohn's disease. Spasm of the puborectalis muscle is noted (*larger arrow*)

Symptoms

About 25% of patients with perianal Crohn's disease are asymtomatic or require no treatment. Pruritus ani and mild discomfort after the passage of stool occur in some patients. When abscesses are present, pain, fever, and systemic symptoms may occur. A system for classification of severity has been developed based on the amount of pain, limitation of activity, restriction of sexual activity, type of perianal involvement, and degree of induration.

Diagnosis

Physical examination reveals enlarged anal skin tags (termed "elephant ears"), perianal openings due to fistulization, induration of the surrounding skin, anal abscesses, and anal strictures. Patients may have complex perianal involvement with ulceration and multiple fistula tracks. Extension to the labia, scrotum, thigh, groin, and buttocks may be present (see Figs. 3.21–3.23). Testing may include the use of CT, magnetic resonance imaging (MRI), anorectal ultrasound, or fistulography as clinically indicated.

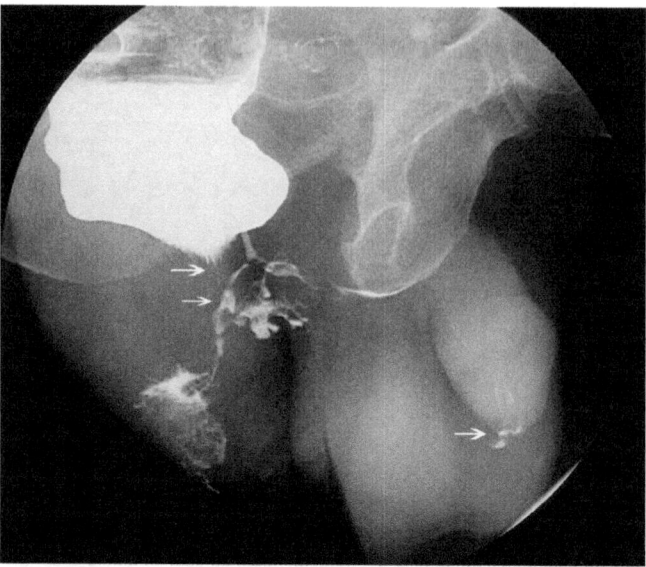

Fig. 3.22 Anal urethral fistula (*arrows*) in a male patient with perianal Crohn's disease. A small quantity of contrast is seen exiting the penis from the urethra (*arrow*)

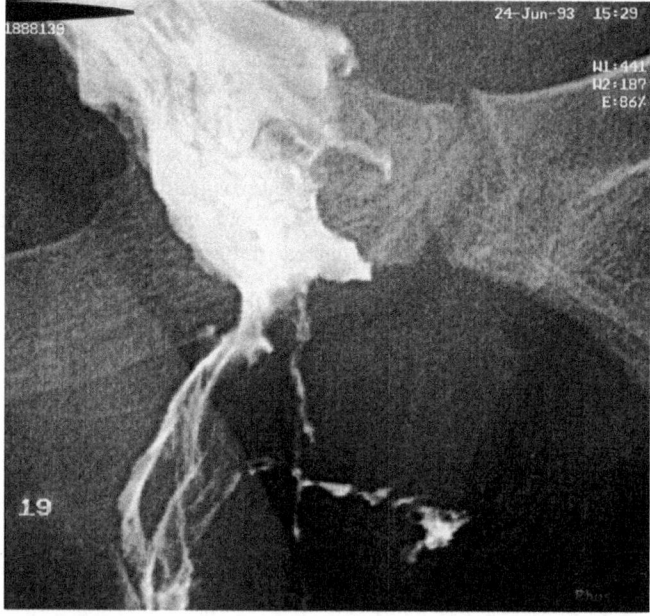

Fig. 3.23 Fistulization from the perianal region to the thigh and gluteal areas in a patient with long-standing Crohn's disease

Treatment

Medical

Medical therapy for Crohn's disease may also be suitable for the perianal complications of the disease. Immunomodulators, including 6-mercaptopurine and azathioprine, may induce healing of perianal disease. Antibiotic therapy, particularly metronidazole has been found to be beneficial. Recently, infliximab (Remicade) has been shown to be highly effective in healing perianal fistulas.

Surgical

Patients with perianal Crohn's disease often require surgery. Surgical management includes incision and drainage of perianal and perirectal abscesses (see Chap. 19), placement of draining devices such as setons, and modified fistulotomy with or without an advancement flap. Some patients with severe perianal Crohn's disease will require a diverting ileostomy or a proctectomy and permanent ileostomy placement (see Chap. 22).

Clinical Pearls

Although rare, perianal carcinoma is a known complication of perianal Crohn's disease. Marked changes in symptomatology should prompt a careful investigation, including possible examination under anesthesia. Fistula surgery must be carefully performed in the setting of active Crohn's disease as prolonged difficulties with wound healing may occur as a complication of surgery. Decisions regarding surgical management depend on the presence or absence of active Crohn's disease in other portions of the bowel, whether Crohn's disease is involving the rectum, and whether complex fistulas are present.

Perianal Fistula

Definition

A pathologic connection between the anal canal and the perianal skin.

Epidemiology

Anal fistulas and abscesses are twice as common in men as in women. Most occur between the ages of 20 and 40 years. Twenty-eight percent of patients with Crohn's disease develop perianal fistulas.

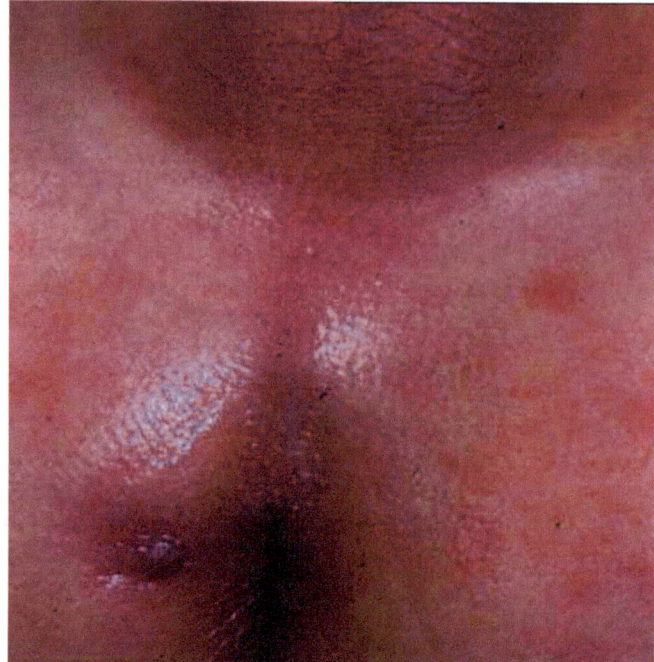

Fig. 3.24 A perianal opening can be clearly visualized as a small papule

Patients at Risk

Patients with Crohn's disease, persons practicing receptive anal intercourse, prior radiation in the perianal region, prior anal surgery, hematologic malignancies, or prior anal trauma.

Symptoms

Drainage of pus, anal irritation, pain with defecation, pruritus ani, bleeding, and the sensation of a swelling or an opening near the anus.

Diagnosis

Physical examination reveals a small external opening with or without drainage (see Figs. 3.24 and 3.25). This may look like a tiny skin lesion. According to Goodsall's rule, an imaginary transverse line should be drawn across the anus, and an external lesion seen anterior to this line opens directly from the anal canal (see Figs. 3.26 and 3.27).

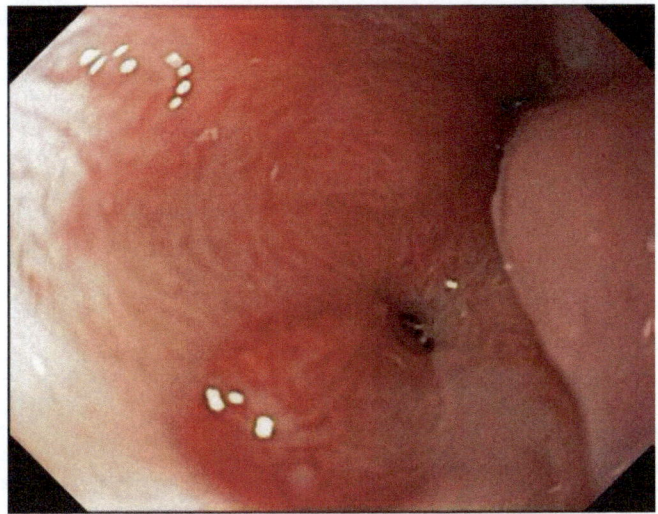

Fig. 3.25 Endoscopic view of fistula in the anal canal

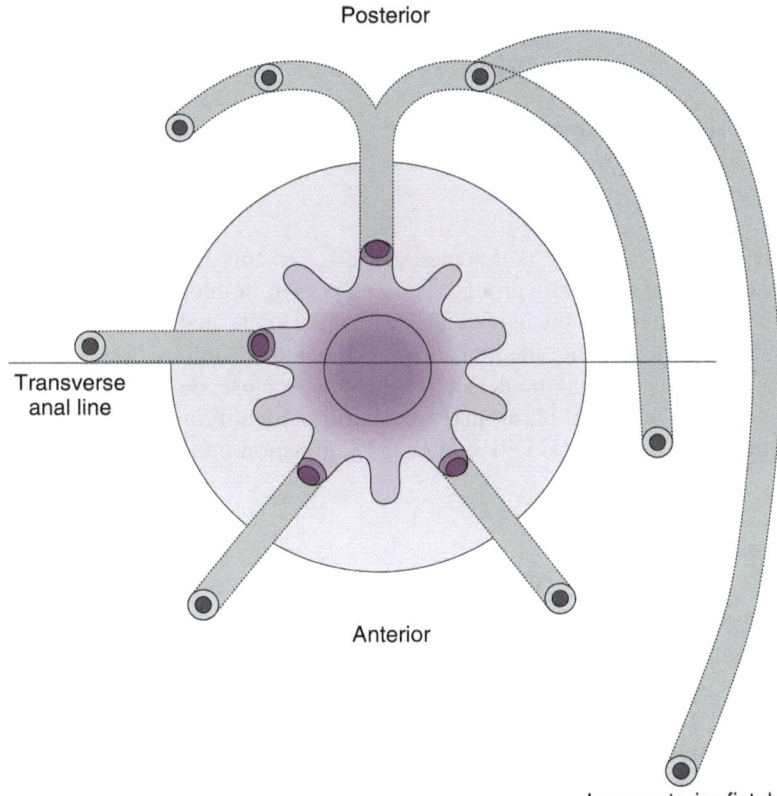

Fig. 3.26 Goodsall's rule for finding the internal opening of an anal fistula based on the location of the external opening. When an imaginary line is drawn through the center of the anus, external openings anterior to the line follow a radial (straight path towards the anal canal). If the external opening is posterior to the line, the fistulous tract will curve and leave the anal canal in the posterior midline

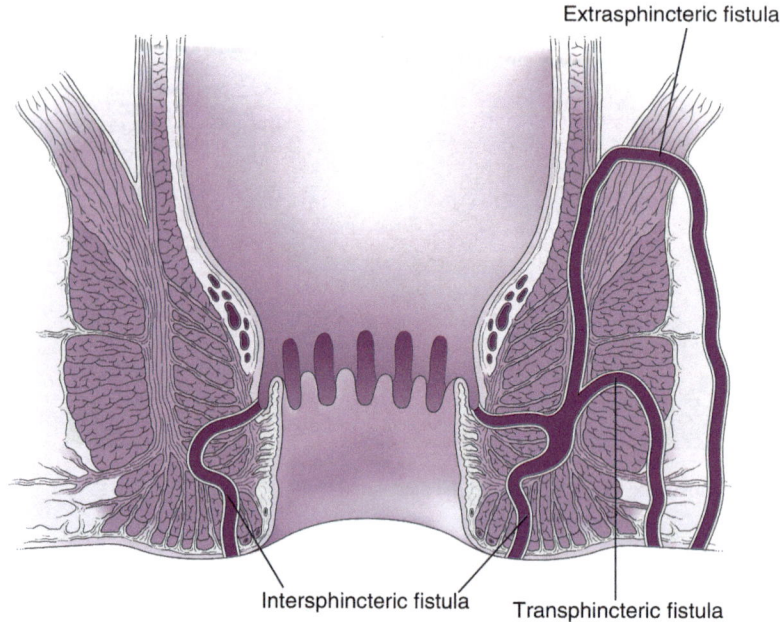

Fig. 3.27 Classification of perinala fistulas

If the external opening is detected posterior to this line, the fistula is more complex and tracks laterally around the anus prior to a midline posterior opening. Bi-digital palpation with the index finger within the anal canal and thumb exterior to the anal canal may enable identification of the entire fistulous track. The internal opening of the fistula may be detectable using a proctoscope or flexible sigmoidoscope. MRI and anorectal ultrasound are helpful in identifying the full extent of fistulous tracks. Some patients will require an examination-under-anesthesia (EUA).

Treatment

Management of perianal fistulas is generally surgical. For low fistulas (internal opening below the puborectalis muscle), fistulotomy or opening of the fistula track (following the insertion of a probe into the external opening) is utilized. High fistulas (internal opening above the puborectalis muscle) often require closure of the internal opening and performance of an advancement flap. Drainage using a seton may also be performed. Some patients will require a diverting stoma following the repair of a high, complex perianal fistula (see Chap. 14).

Clinical Pearls

Conservative management and, if possible, avoidance of surgery are recommended in patients with Crohn's disease and perianal fistulas due to difficulty with wound healing and the possible worsening of clinical symptoms as a result of surgery.

Proctalgia Fugax

Definition

Episodic, intense anal pain of short duration that is unexplainable following thorough evaluation.

Epidemiology

Proctalgia fugax occurs in up to 18% of the population of the United States. It is more common in males and individuals who are less than 40 years of age.

Patients at Risk

Persons with irritable bowel syndrome, anxiety, and stress are at risk. Proctalgia fugax appears to be more common in patients who are perfectionists or hypochondriacs, and those with a family history of proctalgia fugax.

Pathophysiology

Proctalgia fugax appears to be due to a sensory dysfunction, with possible hypersensitivity of the internal anal sphincter and rectal musculature. Stressful events appear to precipitate the occurrence of symptoms.

Symptoms

Proctalgia fugax is defined clinically as the development of sudden, very severe anal pain of very short duration. Pain may last for any length of time from several seconds to 30 min. Intensity of the pain ranges from uncomfortable to unbearable. Associated symptoms may include an extreme urge to defecate, diaphoresis, and presyncope.

Diagnosis

The diagnosis of proctalgia fugax is based on classic symptomatology. Flexible sigmoidoscopy may be performed to rule out other entities.

Treatment

Careful explanation and reassurance about the condition are critical for treatment. A high-fiber diet, Kegel exercises, and psychotherapy may be beneficial. Inhaled salbutamol may be prescribed for immediate pain relief during episodes. A variety of medical therapies have been attempted including nitroglycerin, amyl nitrate, clonidine, antidepressants, and benzodiazepines. Although success has been reported with these treatments, only a small number of patients were included in the groups studied.

Clinical Pearls

The pain associated with proctalgia fugax is similar to the pain associated with levator ani syndrome. Levator ani syndrome is characterized by episodic anorectal pain and intense spasm of the anal muscles. Patients commonly report difficulty with evacuation. Digital rectal examination reveals marked tenderness of the anal sphincter. Anal tenderness on examination is not a feature of proctalgia fugax.

Pruritus Ani

Definition

Itching of the skin around the anus.

Epidemiology

Pruritus ani is more common in males than females and is the most common anorectal complaint presented to dermatologic specialists.

Table 3.2 Causes of pruritis ani

Anorectal disorders	Diarrhea, fecal incontinence
	Hemorrhoids, rectal prolapse
	Fissures, fistulas
	Anal scarring, anal stenosis
	Hidradenitis
	Malignancy, anal cancer, Bowen's disease, and perianal Paget's disease
Infections	Fungal: candidiasis, dematophytes, *Tinea cruris, and* actinomycosis
	Parasitic: pinworms, scabies, lice, and amoebiasis
	Bacterial: *Staphyloccocus aureus*, tuberculosis
	Venereal: herpes, gonorrhea, syphilis, and condyloma acuminatum
Local irritants	Moisture, obesity, and excessive perspiration
	Soaps, hygiene products
	Toilet paper: perfumed, dyed
	Underwear: irritating fabrics, detergents
	Anal creams
	Dietary: coffee, alcohol, acidic foods, chocolate, nuts, and milk
	Drugs: mineral oil, ascorbic acid, quinidine, and colchicine
Dermatologic diseases	Psoriasis, eczema
	Dermatitis (atopic, seborrheic, dermatomyositis)
	Pemphigus
Psychogenic	Anxiety, excessive washing or rubbing of the anal area
	Autoeroticism
Systemic disorders	Diabetes
	Hyperoxaluria, systemic lupus erythematosus
	Liver disease

Patients at Risk

This symptom is usually not associated with the presence of other diseases; however, a large number of conditions can cause pruritus ani (see Table 3.2).

Pathophysiology

Pruritus ani is more common in individuals who have heightened internal anal sphincter relaxation with rectal distention. This may result in irritation of the perianal region from occult leakage of minute amounts of fecal material from the rectum. Excessive rubbing of the skin results in a decrease in thickness of the fatty skin layer, which exacerbates the problem (see Fig. 3.28). Zealous cleansing of the perianal area with alkaline soaps causes contact irritation and dermatitis.

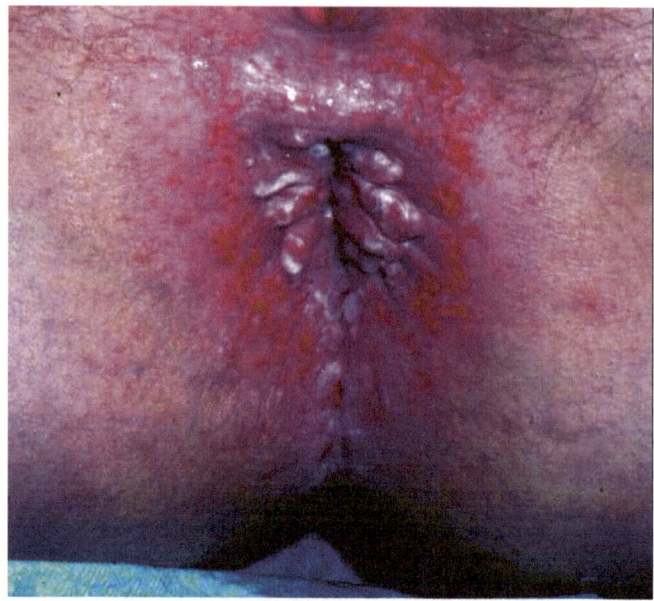

Fig. 3.28 Lichenification of the perianal skin due to recurrent pruritis ani

Symptoms

Itching occurs in the perianal region but may also involve the scrotum or vulva. Symptoms most commonly worsen at night. Little benefit is achieved by scratching the affected area(s) and may worsen the condition.

Diagnosis

Close examination of the perianal region is required. Scrapings to rule out fungal and yeast infection may be helpful. Anoscopy or flexible sigmoidoscopy has been suggested. Some authors recommend the performance of full colonoscopic evalua- tion to rule out colorectal pathology such as Crohn's disease. Perianal skin biopsy may be useful in severe cases.

Treatment

Explanation and reassurance are required to assist with therapy. Dietary manage- ment may be beneficial with temporary elimination of the aforementioned dietary components. Fiber and other bulking agents may also be beneficial. Anal hygiene in the form of cleansing of the perianal region with warm water after each bowel movement is suggested but minimal usage of soap is encouraged. Moistened alcohol free skin wipes that do not contain perfume or witch hazel may be beneficial. Local anesthetic skin ointments are beneficial on an as-needed basis.

Chronic therapy with lubricating agents such as Balneol and Tucks may be effective for refractory cases. Colloidal oatmeal-containing baths may also provide relief. Hydrocortisone containing ointments can be used on a temporary basis (less than 3 months).

Clinical Pearls

Pruritus ani is an extremely common complaint. It is often present in patients who practice excessive anal hygiene, particularly following a bowel movement. In our clinic, patients are advised to carry skin wipes in small containers for use after bowel movements; many patients say this is useful. Some authors have stated that more than 90% of patients who follow the above mentioned treatments develop marked improvement in their condition. Refractory patients should be referred to a dermatologist.

Radiation Proctopathy

Definition

Acute or chronic injury to the rectum (and/or anus) in patients who have received pelvic irradiation.

Epidemiology

Males

There are 180,000 new cases of prostate cancer annually in the United States. Approximately one-third receives radiation therapy.

Females

There are 36,000 new cases of uterine cancer and 12,000 cases of cervical cancer annually in the United States. Approximately one-third receives radiation therapy. Symptoms of acute proctopathy occur in up to 30% of radiation therapy patients. Chronic gastrointestinal symptoms are common (estimates vary from 5 to 47%).

Patients at Risk

Male and female patients undergoing pelvic radiation therapy.

Pathophysiology

Acute Radiation Proctopathy

Epithelial and vascular endothelial cells develop injury following radiation exposure. Symptoms occur during and up to 6 weeks after completion of a course of radiation therapy.

Chronic Radiation Proctopathy

Progressive vascular injury and mucosal epithelial cell destruction occurs. Mucosal atrophy, fibrosis, and secondary telangiectasia formation develops (see Figs. 3.29 and 3.30). Symptoms generally occur 6–12 months after completion of radiation therapy but may be delayed for up to 20 years. Severe complications include rectal ulcerations, stricture formation (see Fig. 3.31), bowel obstruction, fistulization (see Fig. 3.32), and secondary cancer formation.

Symptoms

Acute Radiation Proctopathy

Diarrhea, straining, and urgency.

Chronic Radiation Proctopathy

Rectal bleeding, evacuation difficulty, frequent evacuation, urgency, diarrhea, and fecal incontinence.

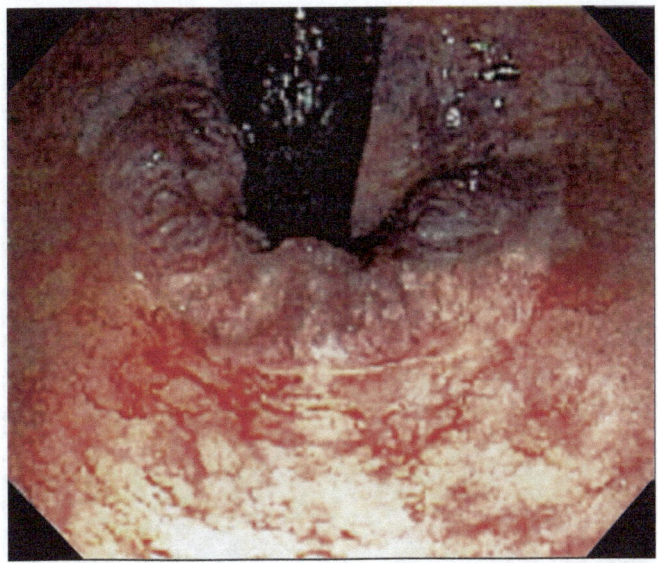

Fig. 3.29 Rectal telangiectasia and internal hemorrhoids seen in a patient with radiation therapy

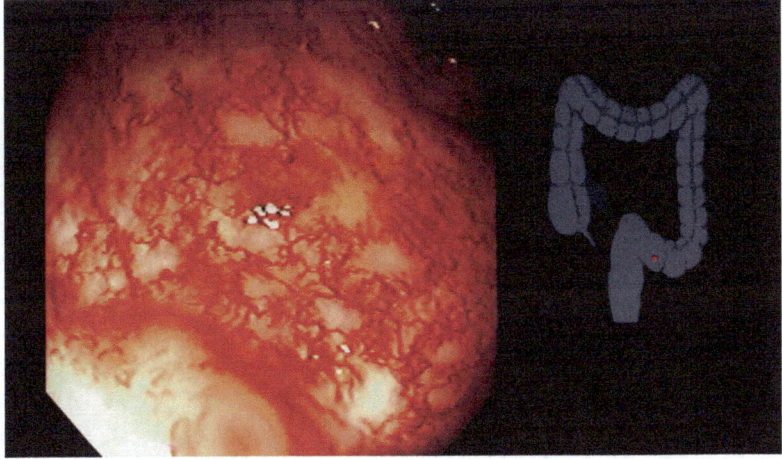

Fig. 3.30 Radiation protography characterized by ischemia and telangiectasia formation. No inflammation is present

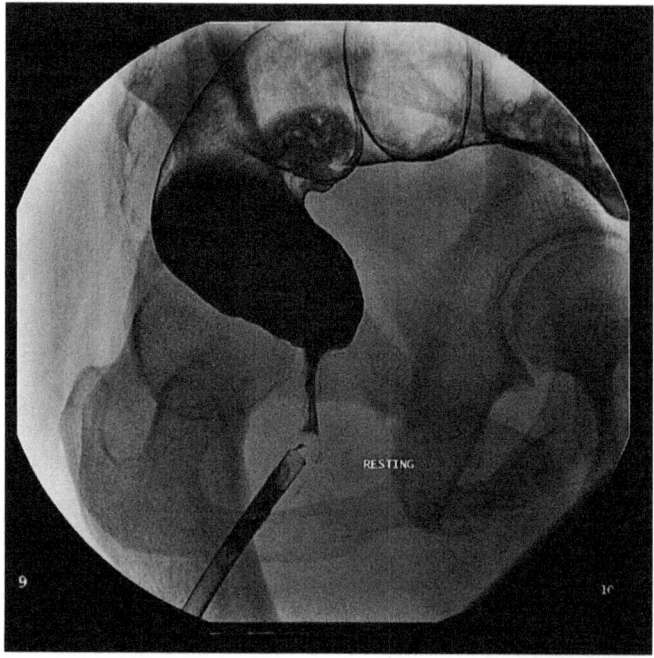

Fig. 3.31 Benign anal stricture in a patient with prior radiation therapy. Tip of catheter is present

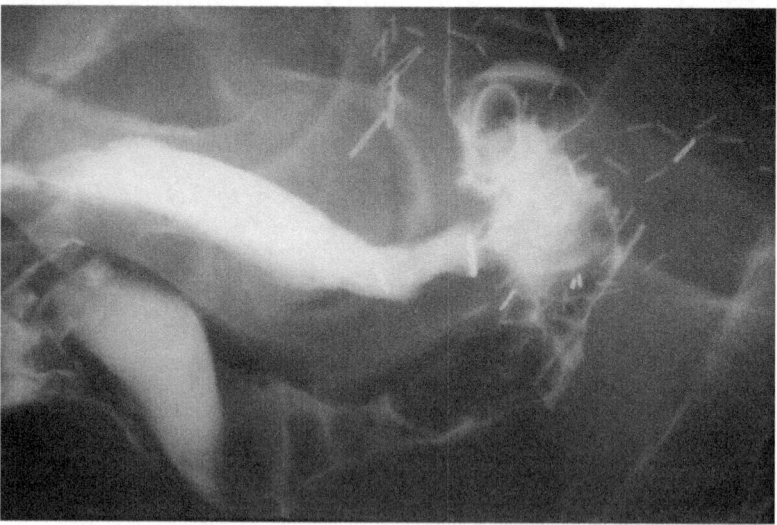

Fig. 3.32 Rectovaginal fistula in a patient with prior radiation therapy for cervical cancer. Copious filling of the vagina with barium is seen

Diagnosis

Flexible sigmoidoscopy to evaluate the affected area. Colonoscopy is indicated for rectal bleeding to rule out other sources.

Treatment

Acute Radiation Proctopathy

Antidiarrheals, a low fiber diet, and change interval of radiation treatment is utilized. The radiation oncologist usually institutes these treatments.

Chronic Radiation Proctopathy

Rectal Bleeding

Endoscopic therapy including laser, argon plasma coagulation, or bipolar electro-cautery is used to obliterate bleeding telangiectasias. Topical formalin application and hyperbaric oxygen therapy may be beneficial. In addition, a role for sucralfate, antioxidants (vitamins C and E), estrogen/progesterone, and corticosteriods has been suggested based on beneficial effects noted in a small number of patients.

Other Associated Symptoms

Sucralfate, short chain fatty acid enemas, corticosteroids, and 5-ASA compounds may be beneficial. Our group has shown that oral retinyl palmitate (8,000 IU b.i.d.) greatly improves these symptoms.

Surgery

Surgery is reserved for refractory bleeding, bowel obstruction, strictures, and fistulization. Surgery consists of formation of a diverting colostomy or proctectomy (see Chap. 22). Formation of a colonic J pouch (see Chap. 18) may be performed in younger patients with normal anal sphincter function.

Clinical Pearls

Radiation proctopathy is a relatively common disorder, that have received very little attention with regard to development of new treatments. It is anticipated that these conditions will be seen with increasing frequency as the population ages and radiation therapy becomes an acceptable alternative to surgical management for prostate cancer and other pelvic malignancies.

Rectal Prolapse

Definition

Displacement of the rectal wall, the anal canal, and the outside of the anus.

Epidemiology

Rectal prolapse is up to 10-times more common in women than in men. It appears to be most common in multiparous women who are over the age of 50 years.

Patients at Risk

Children with cystic fibrosis, spina bifida, congenital neurologic diseases, Marfan's syndrome, and other congenital mesenchymal diseases. Adults with schistosomiasis, spinal cord disorders, and prolapsing pelvic organs such as the uterus and bladder. In addition, patients with chronic constipation and straining and those with rectal or sigmoid tumors.

Pathophysiology

Chronic intussusception of the rectal mucosa appears to initiate the condition. A redundant sigmoid colon and decreased external anal sphincter function are aggravating factors. Long-standing rectal prolapse and straining on the toilet result in damage to pelvic nerves, which exacerbates the problem. Overall weakness of the pelvic floor appears to be another important factor. Rectoanal intussusception is the mildest form of rectal prolapse, and occurs when the rectal mucosa prolapses into (but not outside) the anal canal. Prolapse of the mucosa alone may also occur

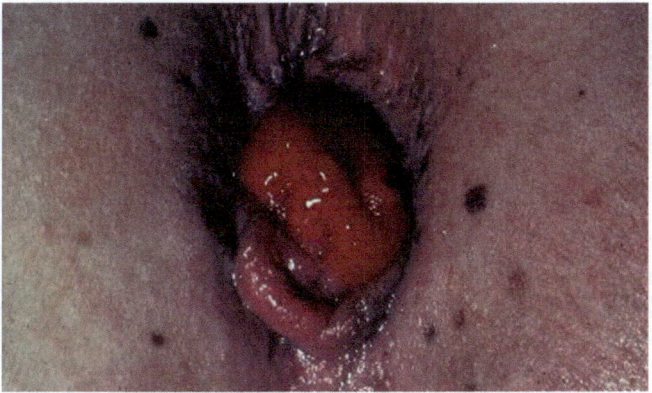

Fig. 3.33 Part of the rectal mucosa has prolapsed a few inches from the anal verge

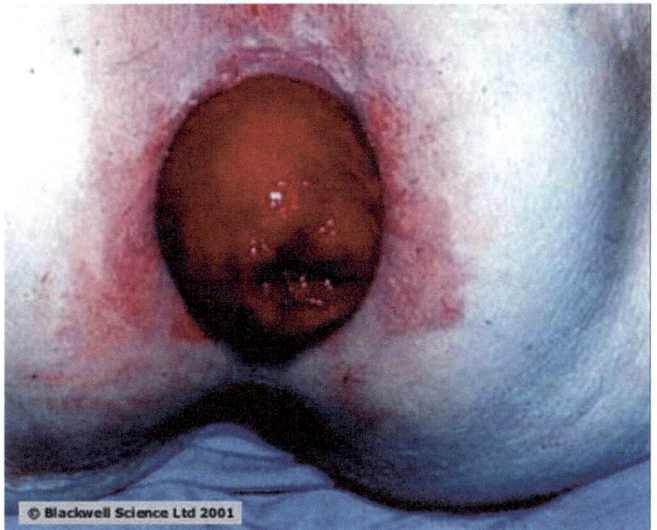

Fig. 3.34 Physical examination of an elderly woman demonstrating a complete rectal prolapse

(see Fig. 3.33). In the most severe forms of rectal prolapse, all portions of the rectal wall protrude outside of the anus (see Fig. 3.34).

Symptoms

Patients will complain of the sensation of a mass protruding from the rectum upon defecation. A long-standing history of straining can often be elicited. Additional symptoms include rectal bleeding, fecal incontinence, pruritus ani,

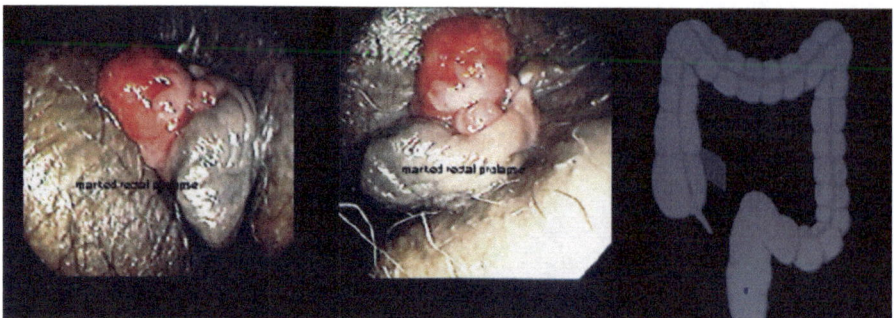

Fig. 3.35 Prolapsed internal hemorrhoid

and rectal pain. In severe cases, inability to reduce the prolapsing rectum and worsening pain may be present. In its most serious form, incarceration of the rectum within and outside of the anal canal may occur with associated ischemia, sepsis, and tissue gangrene.

Diagnosis

Physical examination with maneuvers to increase intraabdominal pressure (such as squatting and straining) will demonstrate a rectal prolapse. Presence of prolapsing mucosal folds differentiates rectal prolapse from prolapsing internal hemorrhoids (see Fig. 3.35). All patients should have an endoscopic evaluation of the colon to rule out a rectal or sigmoid cancer, which may be present in up to 6% of affected patients. Dynamic proctography will document rectoanal intussusception and rectal prolapse not observed on physical examination (see Figs. 3.36 and 3.37).

Treatment

Medical

A complete rectal prolapse is treated with surgery; milder forms may be managed with a high-fiber diet and Sitz™ baths.

Surgical

Surgical approaches include anterior resection of the redundant rectum and sigmoid tissue (which can be performed with a transabdominal or perineal approach).

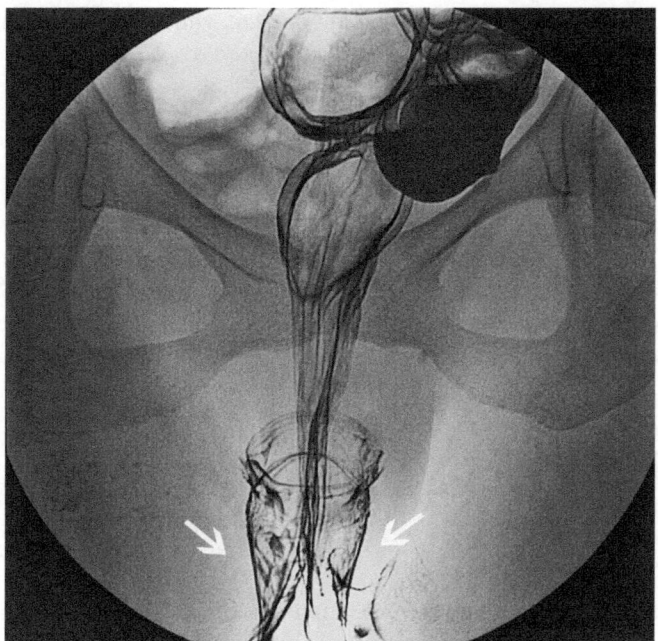

Fig. 3.36 Rectal prolapse (*arrows*) demonstrated on dynamic proctography

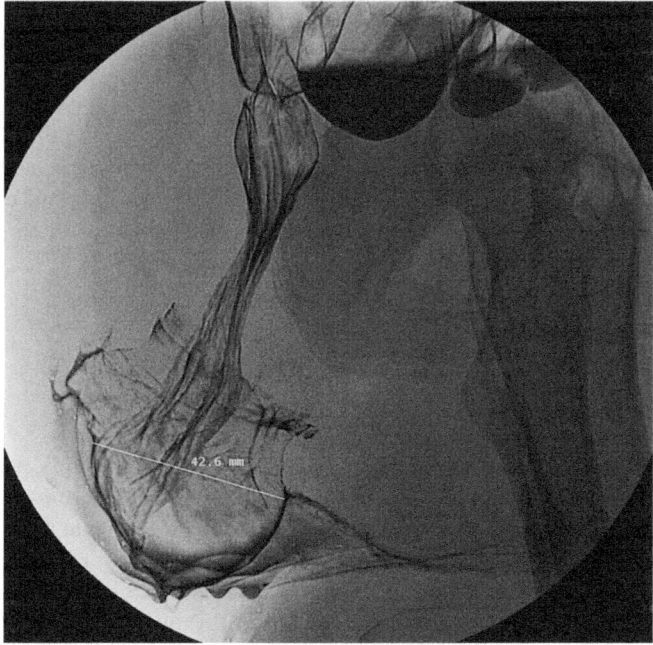

Fig. 3.37 Rectal prolapse demonstrated on dynamic proctography on a patient with chronic constipation. Stretching of rectal mucosa noted

Rectopexy (attachment of the rectum to the sacrum with or without mesh) is considered part of surgical management (see Chap. 15).

Clinical Pearls

Use of PNTML measurements and anorectal manometry (see Chapt. 2) may be beneficial in predicting the functional results of repair of a rectal prolapse. Patients with pudendal nerve damage and/or poor anal sphincter function would be anticipated to have less benefit following surgery for rectal prolapse to improve fecal incontinence.

Rectovaginal Fistula

Epidemiology

Rectovaginal fistula is a relatively uncommon condition, seen in some patients with Crohn's disease and rarely has a congenital malformation. Rectovaginal fistula is also a secondary consequence of a variety of injuries to the rectal and vaginal walls.

Patients at Risk

Rectovaginal fistulas most commonly develop as a consequence of obstetric injuries, lacerations, episiotomies, and vaginal lacerations. Other causes include Crohn's disease, damage from pelvic irradiation, anorectal trauma, sigmoid diverticulitis, surgery of the pelvic region including hysterectomy, anal or rectal carcinoma, and foreign body injuries to the rectum.

Pathophysiology

In Crohn's disease, transmural inflammation of the rectum and anus causes damage to adjacent organs. Associated proteolysis causes tissue destruction and disruption of the normal separation between adjacent organs. Because the anterior wall of the rectum is adjacent to the posterior wall of the vagina, transmural rectal inflammation from Crohn's proctitis results in sinus formation and fistulization (see Fig. 3.38). Obstetric injuries from lacerations may extend from the vagina to the rectal wall. Diverticulitis may cause fistulization from the sigmoid colon to the vagina due to diverticular perforation and local extension of inflammation and infection, particularly

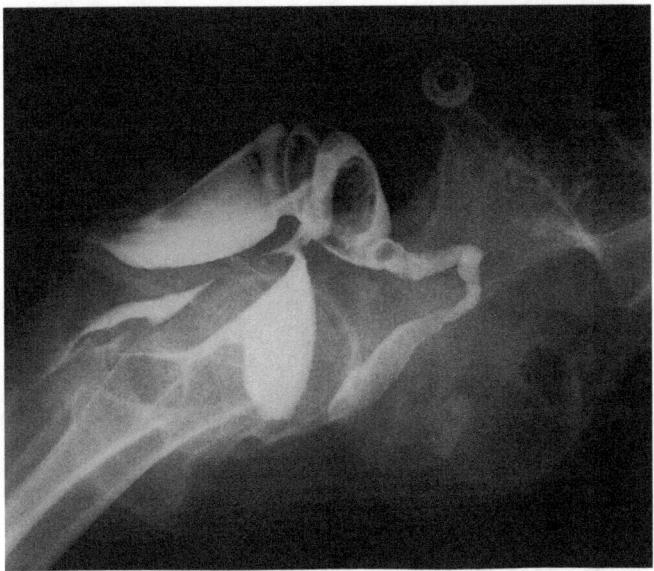

Fig. 3.38 Rectovesicular, rectovaginal, and coloenteric fistula in a patient with Crohn's disease

in patients who have undergone a hysterectomy. Trauma causes either direct penetration between the rectum and vagina or may cause ischemia of either organ, which could lead to fistulization to the other organ during wound healing. Radiation-induced fistulization is generally due to injury to both the rectum and vagina (see Fig. 3.39).

Symptoms

The most common symptoms are the passage of air, feces and/or purulent material from the vagina. Vaginal or rectal bleeding, diarrhea, and fecal incontinence may also occur.

Diagnosis

Physical examination of the anus and vagina occasionally demonstrates a fistula from the anus or the lower portion of the rectum. Identification of the fistula with flexible sigmoidoscopy should be attempted. A barium enema, dynamic proctography, or CT scan may also be useful in visualizing the fistula. If the fistula cannot be identified using these modalities, and the patient has symptoms that are highly suggestive

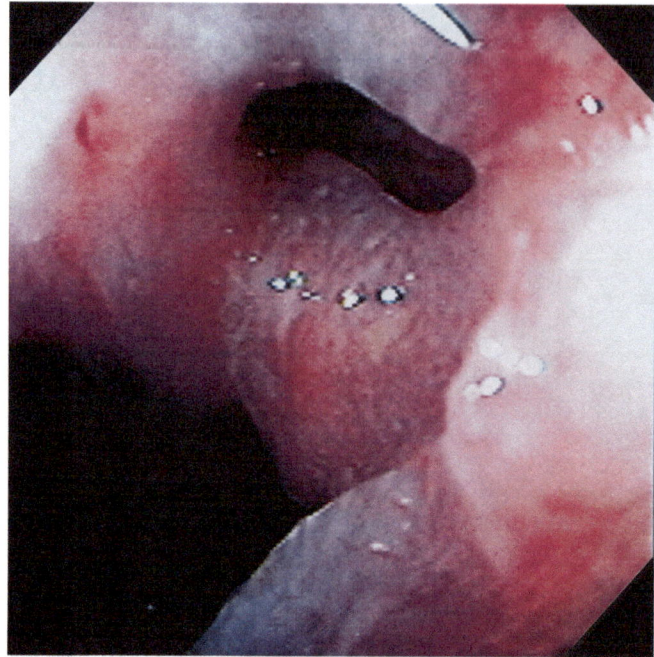

Fig. 3.39 Endoscopic view of a rectovaginal fistula in a patient with prior radiation therapy

of a rectovaginal fistula, demonstration of the fistula may be achieved by placing a tampon in the vagina followed by instillation of 100 mL of methylene blue into the rectum. Instillation of water or saline into the vagina and placement of a sigmoidoscope in the rectum may also be beneficial: air is injected through the sigmoidoscope, and bubbling of air will be seen in the vagina if a fistula is present.

Treatment

Rectovaginal fistulas warrant surgical repair. A variety of operations are performed based on the location of the fistula. Techniques for simple fistula repair include transanal repair, transvaginal repair, or endorectal advancement flap placement. Patients with Crohn's disease or radiation-induced rectovaginal fistulas may require a proctectomy. Some patients with radiation injuries have benefited from muscle flap interposition between the two organs, which improves the rate of successful repair (see Chap. 16).

Clinical Pearls

It is often difficult to identify rectovaginal fistulas in the upper portion of the vagina, particularly in women who have undergone a hysterectomy. In these cases, fistulization occurs at the vaginal cuff. Some of the previously described maneuvers may be required to identify the presence of these fistulas.

Solitary Rectal Ulcer Syndrome

Definition

A disorder characterized by rectal mucosal damage and rectal bleeding with anorectal pain.

Epidemiology

Solitary rectal ulcer syndrome (SRUS) is seen in individuals who strain during defecation. It has also been associated with rectal prolapse, self-digitization, and spastic anorectal disorders such as nonrelaxing puborectalis syndrome.

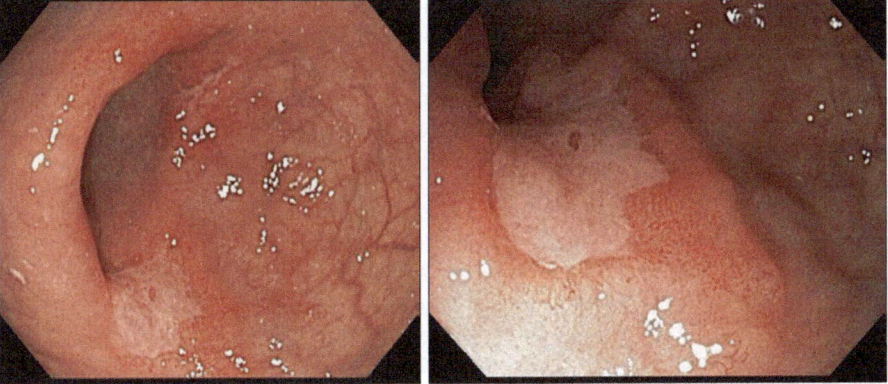

Fig. 3.40 Two endoscopic views of a patient with solitary rectal ulcer syndrome. Two areas of ulceration are seen, as well as erythema involving the second valve of Houston

Patients at Risk

SRUS is more common in female young adults, and is seen in individuals perform-ing manual disimpaction, persons practicing anal autoeroticism, and victims of rape or sexual abuse.

Pathophysiology

SRUS appears to be caused by mucosal ischemia and ulceration. It may be triggered by rectal prolapse causing decreased blood flow. Hamartomatous malformation and congenital duplication of rectal mucosa may be factors contributing to its development. Repeated straining in individuals with nonrelaxing puborectalis syndrome may worsen the condition. Histologically, there is replacement of the lamina propria near the ulcer with collagen and muscle fibers of the muscularis mucosa. Inflammatory changes occur at the site of the ulceration.

Symptoms

The most common symptom of SRUS is rectal bleeding (98%). Constipation, dis-charge of mucus, tenesmus, and pain in the sacrum or perineum also occur. More than 50% of patients will complain of chronic constipation.

Diagnosis

Flexible sigmoidoscopy or colonoscopy is utilized to make a diagnosis. Endoscopically, discrete or multiple ulcerations with surrounding erythema and induration may be seen. Other descriptions include a raised erythematous region, polypoid region, or plaque-like regions. Lesions are most commonly present in the anterior rectal wall, generally 7–10 cm proximal to the anal verge. Biopsies show classic histologic find-ings as described above.

Treatment

Lifestyle

Avoidance of straining, discontinuation of rectal digitation, a high-fiber diet.

Medical

Laxatives and stool softeners may be beneficial. Sucralfate and hydrocortisone enemas have been suggested but are unproven therapies.

Surgical

Rectopexy before repair of rectal prolapse, insertion of a perianal nylon loop, and myotomy of the puborectalis muscle in cases of nonrelaxing puborectalis syndrome. Colostomy may be indicated in cases of severe rectal bleeding (see Chap. 15).

Clinical Pearls

SRUS is frequently misdiagnosed and confused with other conditions such as inflammatory bowel disease and rectal masses such as villous adenoma.

Ulcerative Proctitis

Definition

A chronic inflammatory bowel disorder only affecting the rectum.

Epidemiology

The epidemiology of ulcerative proctitis is similar to ulcerative colitis. Approximately 40% of patients with ulcerative colitis only have manifestations of the disease in the rectum or rectosigmoid colon. Ulcerative colitis occurs throughout the world but is most common in the white population of the United States. Ulcerative colitis is especially common in Jews of Eastern European origin. A number of factors have been identified that appear to predispose to the condition: the ethnic and racial distribution of ulcerative colitis suggests a genetic component of the disorder; environmental factors also play a role. For example, prior appendectomy protects against ulcerative colitis. Additionally, ulcerative colitis is more common in former tobacco smokers and nonsmokers than in current tobacco users.

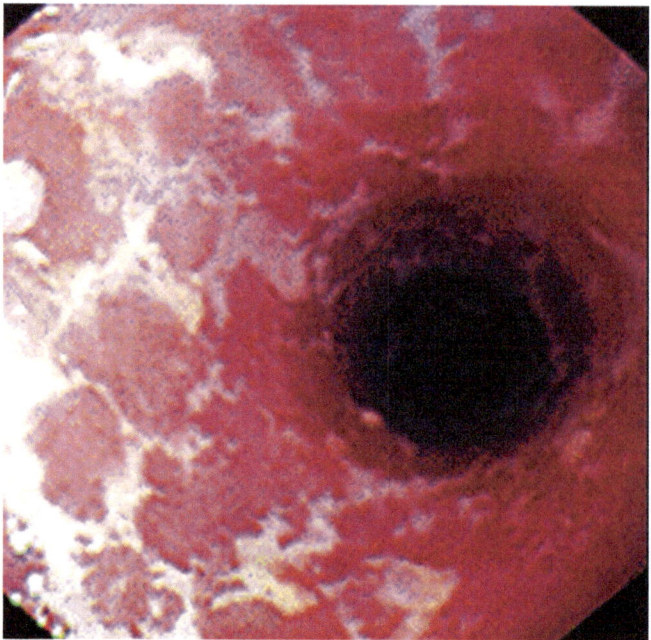

Fig. 3.41 Endoscopic view of moderate colitis demonstrating ulceration, exudates, and loss of vascular pattern of mucosa

Pathophysiology

The mechanism for the development of ulcerative proctitis is similar to that of ulcerative colitis. It is an autoimmune condition characterized by the presence of antibodies to various components of the gastrointestinal mucosa. Cytotoxic T-cell function appears to be enhanced, most likely in response to elevated inflammatory cytokines. Activation of monocytes and T-cells causes increased secretion of a variety of cytokines including tumor necrosis factor, interleukin-1, and interleukin-6.

Endoscopically, the disease is characterized by the presence of mucosal inflammation beginning at the anal verge and extending without interruption in a proximal fashion. This is in contrast to Crohn's disease, which commonly spares the rectum and is characterized by "skip areas" of normal mucosa between inflamed portions of the bowel. Depending on the severity of the inflammation, erythema, edema, granularity, friable hemorrhagic mucosa, loss of normal vascular pattern, punctate ulcerations, larger deep ulcerations, and advanced disease with complete denuding of the mucosa may be seen (see Fig. 3.41). Long-standing ulcerative colitis may be characterized by chronic stricture formation; however, the presence of a stricture in a patient with ulcerative colitis should raise concern that a secondary carcinoma may have developed.

Microscopically, mucosal inflammation is seen with edema and hemorrhage in the lamina propria. Mucosal infiltration with a variety of inflammatory cells

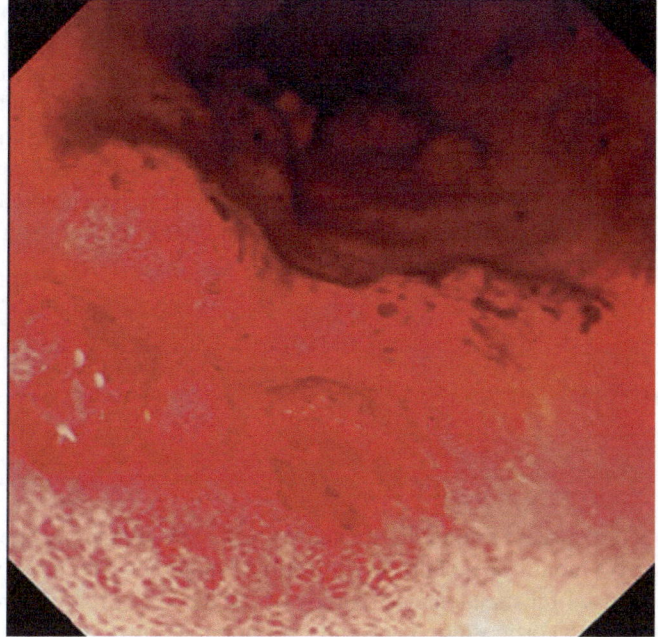

Fig. 3.42 Typical endoscopic appearance of a dysplasia-associated lesion or mass (DALM) in ulcerative colitis

produces cryptitis and crypt abscess formation. Long-standing ulcerative colitis may result in the development of dysplasia and secondary carcinoma (see Fig. 3.42); however, this appears to be less common in patients with proctitis alone.

Symptoms

The most common symptoms of ulcerative colitis are diarrhea and rectal bleeding. Patients with ulcerative proctitis and left-sided ulcerative colitis often have symptoms of rectal urgency, incomplete evacuation, tenesmus, and, occasionally, fecal incontinence. More severe disease is characterized by systemic symptoms including fever, weight loss, and signs and symptoms of anemia.

Diagnosis

Sigmoidoscopy is generally utilized to make the initial diagnosis of ulcerative colitis and ulcerative proctitis. Careful description of the findings on sigmoidoscopy is recommended to indicate the endoscopic severity of the disease. Biopsies are obtained to diagnose ulcerative colitis and to rule out other forms of colitis including infectious colitis, ischemic colitis, pseudomembranous colitis, and nonsteroidal anti-inflammatory drug-induced colitis. Because rectal bleeding and changing bowel habits may indicate the presence of other diseases such as colonic malignancy, evaluation of the entire colon with a colonoscopy may be required if typical symptoms of colitis are not revealed on sigmoidoscopy. Colonoscopy is also used to determine the extent of colonic involvement and endoscopic severity of the disease.

Treatment

Medical

Mild to moderate disease is initially treated with 5-ASA-containing agents administered either by mouth or rectally in the form of a suppository or enema. These drugs are also used for maintenance therapy of the disease. More severe cases are treated acutely with corticosteroids given either parenterally, orally, or into the rectum. Patients requiring repeated courses of corticosteroid treatment are started on immune-modulating agents (so-called steroid-sparing drugs) such as azathioprine and 6-mercaptopurine. Typical doses for treatment are as follows:

Acute colitis (severe): prednisone 40–60 mg/day with dose tapering following relief of symptoms. Hospitalized patients are treated with methylprednisolone 40 mg/day by continuous intravenous (IV) drip, or 15 mg IV piggyback (IVBP) 4 times/day.

Acute colitis (mild to moderate) and maintenance therapy: oral mesalamine 2.4–4 g/day. A variety of forms of mesalamine are available on the market. These vary in their release properties and the vehicle that is utilized to prevent the destruction of mesalamine prior to delivery to the appropriate inflamed portions of the gastrointestinal tract. Mesalamine suppositories (500 mg dose) are administered once or twice today. Mesalamine retention enemas are given as a single 4 g (60 mL) dose that is retained for 8 h at night. Recommended doses of azathioprine and 6-mercaptopurine (which are generally reserved for maintenance therapy in patients requiring repeated corticosteroid treatment) are 2.5 and 1.5 mg/kg/day, respectively.

Surgical

Surgery is indicated for acute disease that is refractory to IV corticosteroid therapy (or cyclosporine in some centers), or complicated by perforation or toxic megacolon. Surgery is also indicated for chronic poorly controlled disease, and the secondary development of cancer, precancerous lesions, or dysplasia.

Total proctocolectomy is the surgical treatment of choice for ulcerative colitis. In elderly patients, or patients who are unable to undergo further surgery, a permanent Brook ileostomy is performed. In younger patients with intact anal sphincter functions an ileoanal anastomosis and creation of an ileal pouch (also known as a J pouch) will be performed (see Chap. 17). Surgeries are most commonly recommended for patients with pancolitis (involving the entire colon). It is very uncommon for patients with ulcerative proctitis alone to require surgical therapy.

Clinical Pearls

Recent studies, including meta-analyses of the medical literature, indicate that therapy with topical mesalamine is more effective than oral mesalamine in the treatment of acute ulcerative proctitis and for maintenance therapy of the disease.

Since the risk of colon cancer increases dramatically in patients who have had ulcerative colitis for more than 10 years, regular surveillance colonoscopy with multiple mucosal biopsies throughout the colon is performed annually.

Surveillance colonoscopy is recommended every 2–3 years in patients with isolated ulcerative proctitis.

Chapter 4
Neoplasms of the Anus

Eli D. Ehrenpreis

Anal Carcinoma

Tumor Subtypes

Cloacal

Cloacal tumors arise from the transitional epithelium lined zone separating the rectum from the squamous-lined portion of the anal canal proximal to the dentate line.

Squamous Cell

Squamous cell tumors arise from the squamous epithelium in the anal canal.

Perianal Skin and Anal Margin Tumors

These tumors arise from keratinized, hair-bearing skin near the entrance of the anal canal (see Fig. 4.1).

E.D. Ehrenpreis, MD (✉)
Chief of Gastroenterology and Endoscopy, Highland Park Hospital,
NorthShore University Health System, Highland Park, IL 60035, USA

Clinical Associate Professor of Medicine, University of Chicago Medical Center,
Highland Park, IL 60035, USA
e-mail: ehrenpreis@gipharm.net

E.D. Ehrenpreis et al. (eds.), *Anal and Rectal Diseases: A Concise Manual*,
DOI 10.1007/978-1-4614-1102-4_4, © Springer Science+Business Media, LLC 2012

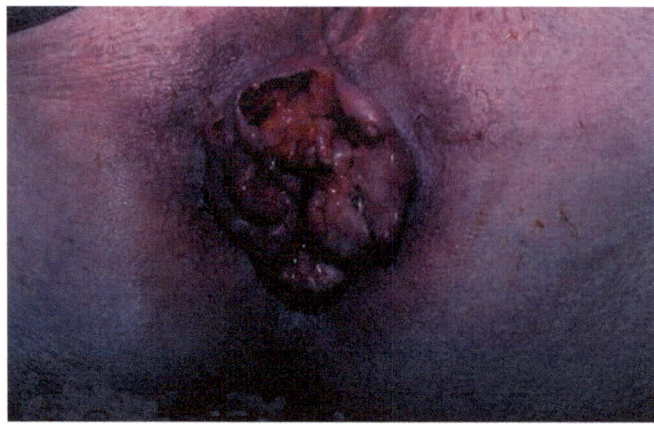

Fig. 4.1 A large anal tumor with ulcerating components is seen on external examination in this elderly female

Epidemiology

The average age of presentation is 57 years. Anal canal tumors are more common in women (60%), whereas perianal skin and anal margin tumors are more common in men (80%).

Patients at Risk

Homosexual men; people who practice receptive anal intercourse; people infected with HIV or human papillomavirus (HPV); people with anal condylomata, cervical cancer, chronic anal fistula, a prior history of syphilis, a prior infection with herpes simplex virus type II, or perianal Crohn's disease; people who have undergone anal irradiation or renal transplantation; and people who smoke.

Symptoms

The most common symptoms are rectal bleeding and pain in the anorectal region; however, 75% of patients are asymptomatic. Pruritus ani, a sensation of fullness or a lump in the anal region, anal discharge, a change in bowel habits, or pain in the pelvic region may occur.

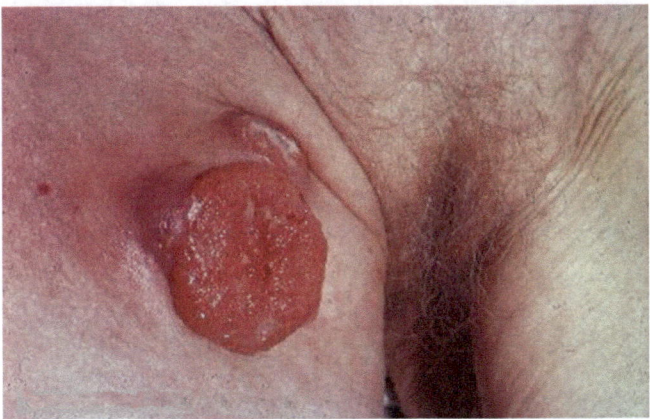

Fig. 4.2 Anal carcinoma with secondary inguinal lymph node deposit

Pathophysiology

A strong relationship exists between anal and genital HPV infection and the development of anal carcinoma. It is assumed that previous infection with HPV places individuals at risk for the condition. Environmental factors such as cigarette smoking and exposure to other sexually transmitted diseases appear to be important variables. Finally, immunosuppression appears to further promote carcinogenesis.

Diagnosis

Visual inspection is performed initially (see Fig. 4.2). In addition, digital rectal exam, anoscopy, sigmoidoscopy, or a barium study may be performed (see Fig. 4.3). Anesthesia is often required for full evaluation. Diagnosis is made by biopsy of the lesion.

Treatment

Surgical

If the lesion is small, involving only the mucosa and submucosa, a wide local excision is performed. Large, advanced lesions require an abdominoperineal resection and colostomy formation (see Chap. 22).

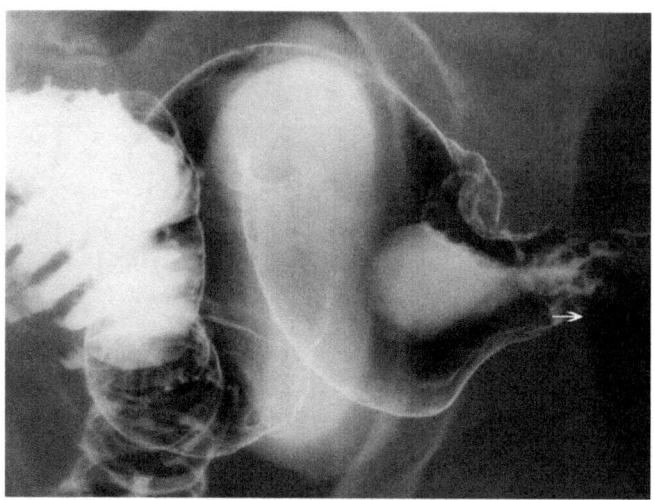

Fig. 4.3 Barium study demonstrates irregular appearance of a lesion (*arrow*)

Combination Radiation and Chemotherapy (The Nigro Protocol)

External beam radiation (30 Gy) is administered over a 3-week period. Concomitant 5-fluorouracil is administered continuously for the first 4 days and again on days 29–32. Mitomycin-C is also given on the first day of treatment. An 85% success rate is expected, and most patients undergoing the Nigro protocol will not require an abdominal–perineal resection or colostomy.

Clinical Pearls

Patients undergoing the Nigro protocol should receive frequent follow-up examinations and biopsies of the anorectal region to evaluate for recurrence. Occasionally, carcinoma of the anus will be discovered in a hemorrhoidectomy specimen. These patients also require surveillance. Some have suggested that patients with perianal or genital condyloma and other forms of HPV infection should undergo routine surveillance for anal carcinoma.

Other Anal Malignancies

Anal Adenocarcinoma

Symptoms

The most common symptoms are anal pain, bleeding, sensation of a mass, and fistula drainage.

Pathophysiology

This is a rare tumor that arises from anal glandular tissue. It is often seen developing in anorectal fistulas.

Diagnosis

Physical examination, anoscopy, and/or flexible sigmoidoscopy.

Treatment

Treatment is usually surgical, the most common procedure being abdominoperineal resection.

Prognosis

The recurrence rate after surgery is very high (54%), and estimated mean survival is between 2 and 3 years. Due to this high rate of recurrence, some investigators have recommended preoperative chemotherapy and radiation therapy.

Basal Cell Carcinoma of the Perianal Region

Epidemiology

This is a rare location for basal cell carcinoma and is stated to represent less than 0.1% of all cases of anorectal tumors. It is more common in men and generally occurs after the age of 50 years.

Symptoms

The most common symptoms are bleeding, ulceration, or a lump-like sensation in the perianal region.

Pathophysiology

This tumor arises from the basal cells of the perianal skin.

Diagnosis

This tumor classically appears as an exophytic lesion (a neoplasm or lesion that grows outward from an epithelial surface) with rolled edges and a central ulceration.

Treatment

These lesions are treated with local incision, sometimes in combination with radiation therapy.

Prognosis

Local recurrences occur in 29% of patients and the 5-year survival rate is 73%.

Bowen's Disease

Epidemiology

This is a rare intraepidermal squamous cell carcinoma.

Pathophysiology

Bowen's disease appears to be a marker for the development of other carcinomas including bronchogenic carcinoma, genitourinary tumors, and gastrointestinal adenocarcinoma.

Diagnosis

It is a slow-growing tumor that is rarely invasive.

Treatment

The lesion is treated with local wide incision.

Malignant Melanoma

Epidemiology

This is a rare tumor that accounts for 0.5–1% of all anal cancers and 0.2–1.6% of all melanomas. Anal melanoma appears to be more than twice as common in women as in men.

Pathophysiology

This tumor arises from melanocytes in the squamous mucosa of the anal canal and possibly the lower rectum.

Symptoms

The most common symptoms are pain, a lump-like sensation in the anal region, constipation and evacuation difficulty, and change in bowel habits. Anorectal bleeding may also occur.

Diagnostic Testing

Physical examination with visualization of the external perianal region is often sufficient to identify the lesion. Lesions higher in the anal canal or in the lower rectum will be seen on flexible sigmoidoscopy or anoscopy.

Treatment

Surgical resection is required. It appears that local resection has the same overall prognosis as radical resection. Adjuvant chemotherapy and radiation therapy have not been proven to be beneficial.

Prognosis

Very poor; 5-year survival has been estimated to be between 0 and 5%.

Perianal Paget's Disease

Epidemiology

This is a rare disorder that resembles Paget's disease of the breast. Average age at diagnosis is approximately 60 years.

Symptoms

Rectal bleeding, discharge, pruritus ani, and pain.

Pathophysiology

Perianal Paget's disease is characterized histologically as a dermatosis with multiple large vascular cells present within the epithelium. Histologically, the cells resemble those of Bowen's disease and are differentiated by positive periodic acid-Schiff staining. Perianal Paget's disease is closely associated with the presence of carcinoma of the anus and rectum.

Diagnosis

Physical examination reveals an erythematous plaque with crusting and scaling.

Treatment

Treatment may include topical retinoid therapy, local surgical resection, and abdominoperineal resection depending on the stage of the disease.

Prognosis

The majority (<75%) of patients with perianal Paget's disease have an adjacent anal carcinoma. Five-year survival has been estimated at about 50%.

Chapter 5
Neoplasms of the Rectum

Eli D. Ehrenpreis

Rectal Carcinoma

Epidemiology

Rectal carcinoma occurs most commonly in patients between 50 and 70 years of age. It is equally common in males and females.

Patients at Risk

Patients with sporadic adenomatous colonic polyps, familial polyposis coli, long-standing ulcerative colitis, a family history of colorectal polyps and colorectal cancers, long-standing Crohn's colitis, or presence of a ureteral diversion colostomy. Other risks include prior radiation therapy, long-standing use of stimulant laxatives, and cholecystectomy.

Pathophysiology

Mutations of oncogenes—genes that transform normal cells into abnormally proliferating cells—are commonly seen in colorectal cancers and large adenomas. Abnormalities in a variety of tumor suppressor genes including deleted in colon

E.D. Ehrenpreis, MD (✉)
Chief of Gastroenterology and Endoscopy, Highland Park Hospital,
NorthShore University Health System, Highland Park, IL 60035, USA

Clinical Associate Professor of Medicine, University of Chicago Medical Center,
Highland Park, IL 60035, USA
e-mail: ehrenpreis@gipharm.net

E.D. Ehrenpreis et al. (eds.), *Anal and Rectal Diseases: A Concise Manual*,
DOI 10.1007/978-1-4614-1102-4_5, © Springer Science+Business Media, LLC 2012

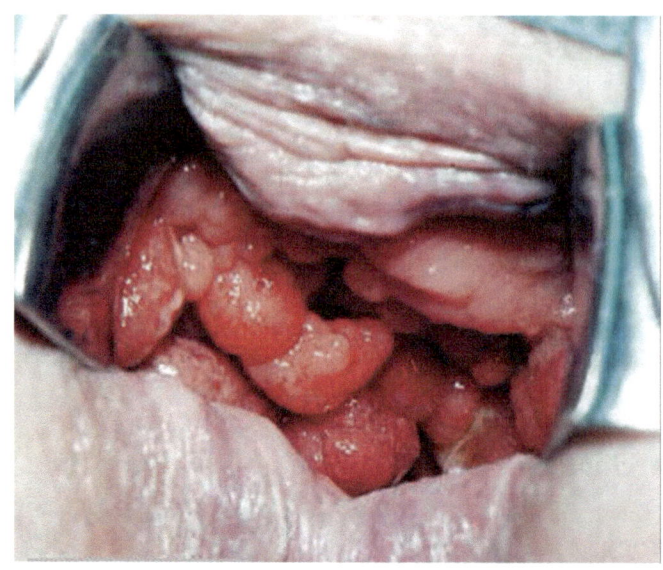

Fig. 5.1 A 24-year-old woman with familial APC has numerous polyps in the rectum, some of which have prolapsed, as seen on sigmoidoscopy

cancer (*DCC*), familial adenomatous polyposis coli (*APC*) gene, *MSH2*, *MLH1*, *PMS1*, *PMS2*, and *MSH6* (hereditary nonpolyposis colorectal cancer genes) have been identified. Patients with APC, an autosomal dominant disease defined by the presence of at least 100 adenomatous polyps within the colon, develop colorectal cancers by the age of 40 years (see Fig. 5.1). The mutated APC gene, located on chromosome 5, has been isolated in this patient group.

Colorectal cancers generally begin as aberrant crypt foci and develop into adenomatous polyps (see Figs. 5.2–5.4). Dysplasia within these lesions becomes more frequent as the size of the polyps increases.

Tubulovillous and villous adenomatous polyps are more likely to have associated dysplasia or intramucosal carcinoma than tubular adenomas. The prevalence of colonic adenomas appears to be about 25% in persons over the age of 50 years.

Environmental factors clearly play a role in the development of colorectal polyps and cancer. The prevalence of colorectal cancer in industrialized countries ranges from 10 to 35 per 100,000 people, while prevalence in Third World countries ranges from 0.2 to 10 per 100,000 people. People from countries with a low prevalence of colorectal carcinoma who move to countries with a high prevalence, for example, Japanese people who have moved to Hawaii, have a much higher prevalence of colorectal cancer than natives of the low prevalence population. High-fat, low fiber diets have been implicated in the increased incidence of colorectal cancer. Obesity and a decrease in activity also appear to play a role.

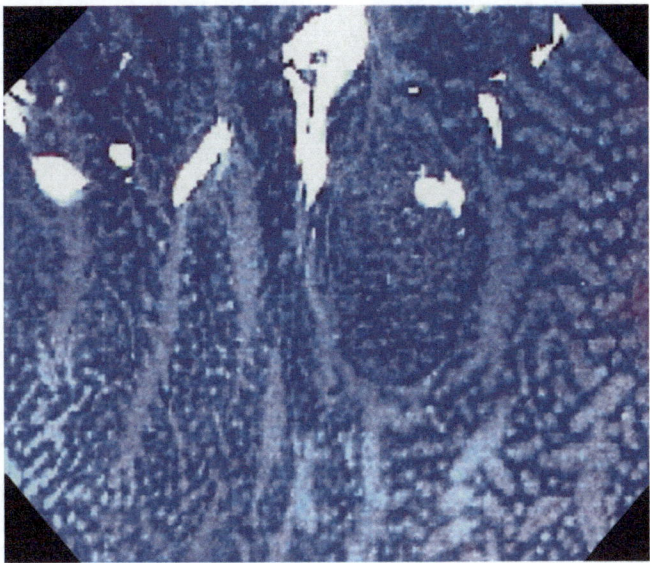

Fig. 5.2 Magnified view of the colonic mucosa stained with methylene blue demonstrating an aberrant crypt locus, a possible precursor of adenomatous tissue (photo courtesy of Dr. Gregory Cohen)

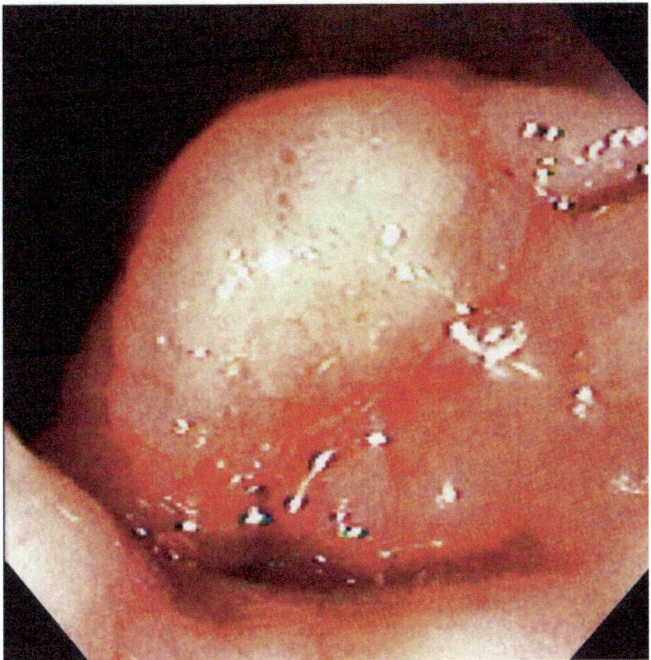

Fig. 5.3 Sessile rectal polyp determined to contain invasive adenocarcinoma

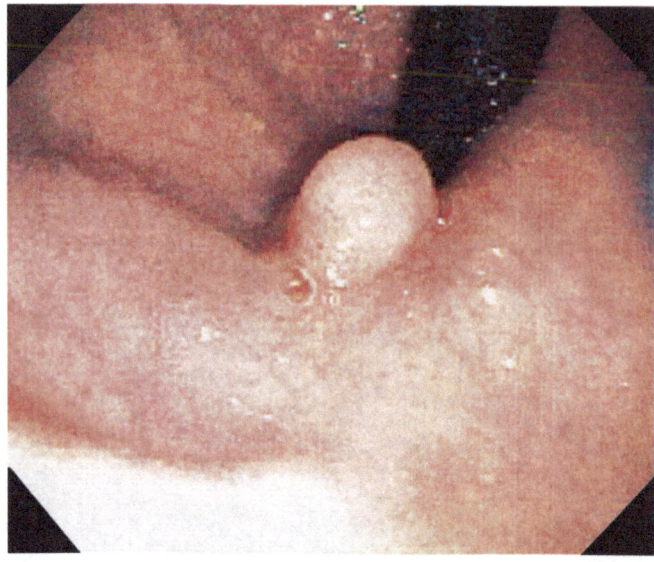

Fig. 5.4 A sessile polyp near the dentate line seen on retroflexion during colonoscopy

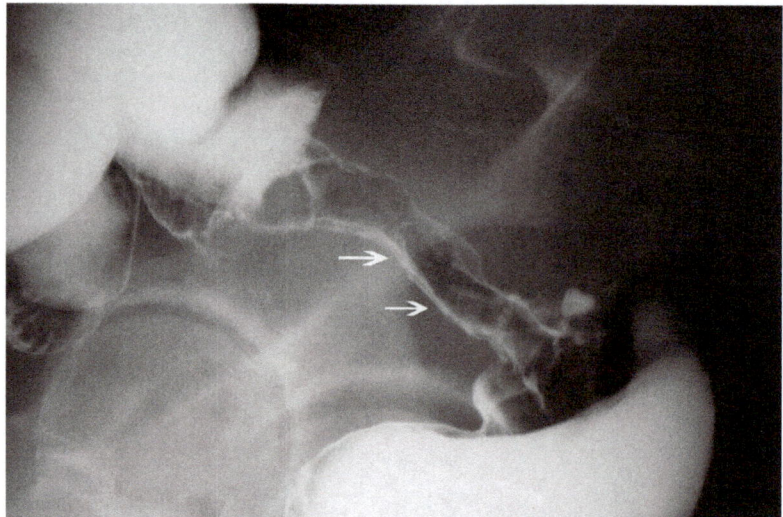

Fig. 5.5 Advanced rectal carcinoma. Lateral view on barium study shows large "apple core" lesions (*arrows*)

Symptoms

Approximately 50% of rectal cancers are asymptomatic at the time of diagnosis. More advanced lesions present with rectal bleeding, change in bowel habits, constipation, obstipation, tenesmus, and passage of thin, narrow stools (see Fig. 5.5). Very advanced lesions may present with the signs and symptoms of iron deficiency anemia, rectal pain, rectal obstruction, weight loss and malaise, colonic perforation, or the signs and symptoms of metastatic disease.

Diagnosis

Digital rectal examination may result in palpation of the lesion (generally if it is within 10 cm of the anal verge). Testing of the stool may reveal the presence of occult blood. Proctoscopy, flexible sigmoidoscopy, or endoscopy is used to visualize the lesion and to obtain biopsies (see Figs. 5.6–5.7). Full colonoscopy is utilized to evaluate for synchronous colorectal neoplasms.

CT scanning and endoscopic ultrasound may be utilized (see Fig. 5.8).

Treatment

In lesions that are restricted to the mucosa, transanal resection with excision of surrounding normal mucosa may be utilized. Endoscopic mucosal resection has

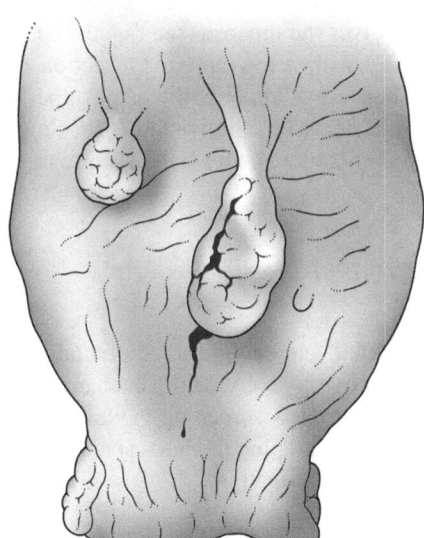

Fig. 5.6 Pedunculated rectal polyps as seen on endoscopy

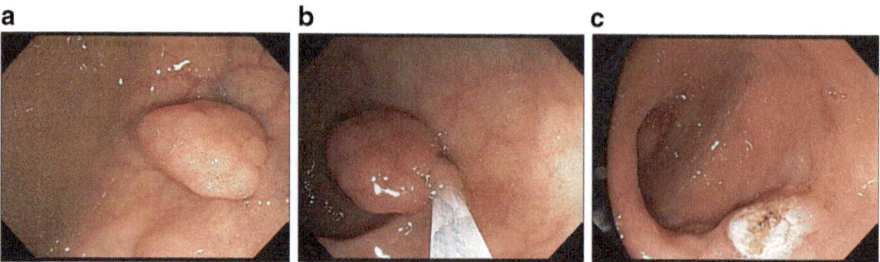

Fig. 5.7 (**a**) Sessile polyp of the rectum. (**b**) Polypectomy technique performed by creating a pseudostalk using a snare technique. (**c**) After electrocautery and removal of the polyp

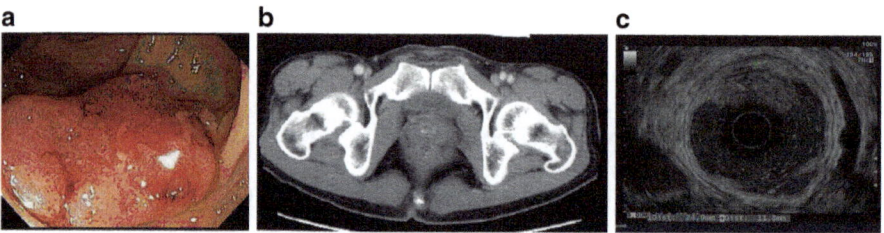

Fig. 5.8 (**a**) Endoscopic view of the large rectal polypoid mass. (**b**) CT unable to differentiate the different rectal layers and extent of invasion. (**c**) EUS delineating the various layers with involvement of the submucosa and invasion of, but not through, the muscularis propria underneath which is seen intact all around as the thin black line (hypoechoic). This was confirmed after low anterior resection as T2N0 rectal adenocarcinoma. Photographs courtesy of Dr. Shailesh Bajaj

recently been advocated as an alternative treatment for rectal cancer that only involves the mucosa (see Fig. 5.9). Larger, more advanced lesions are treated surgically with a low anterior resection or an abdominoperineal resection (APR) (see Chap. 21). Preoperative or postoperative radiation therapy and chemotherapy are indicated with curative intent for stage II and III cancer, and are indicated for palliation in patients with stage IV disease (see Staging of Rectal Cancer).

Clinical Pearls

Regular screening for colorectal neoplasms with full colonic evaluation using colonoscopy has recently been approved in the United States for patients of 50 years or older. New screening methods, including the use of stool-based molecular tests and radiographic methods such as computed tomography colonography, are undergoing investigation.

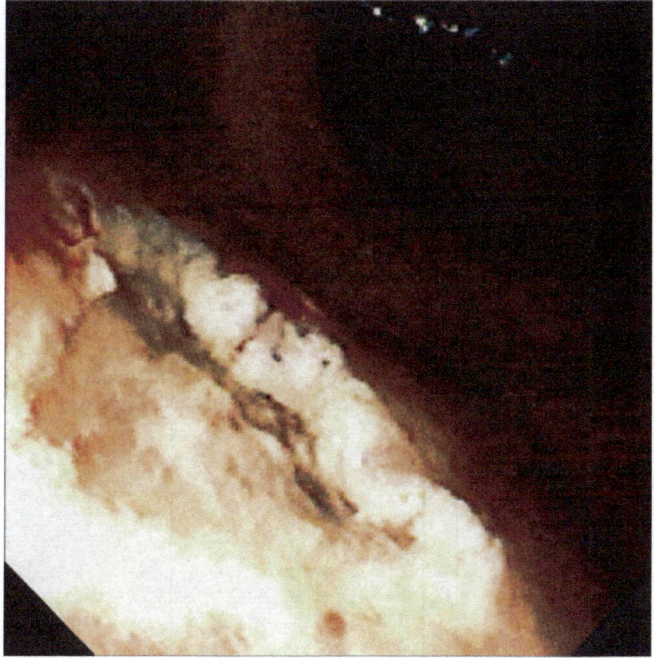

Fig. 5.9 Sessile rectal polyp determined to contain invasive adenocarcinoma as seen after endo-scopic mucosal resection (photo courtesy of Dr. Charles Dye)

Staging of Rectal Cancer

Modified Dukes' Classification

The purpose of staging colorectal cancers is to determine appropriate therapies for individual patients and to establish the prognosis for each case. Specifically, staging helps to determine whether adjuvant chemotherapy and radiation therapy should be utilized in an attempt to cure the disease. The Dukes' classification system was originally established in the 1930s (see Table 5.1). It is based on the depth of tumor penetration and the presence or absence of lymph node involvement. The 5-year survival following surgery in patients who were deemed potentially curable is listed with each stage (for colon and rectal cancer).

Table 5.1 Dukes' classification of adenocarcinoma of the colon or rectum

Classification	Stage A	Stage B1	Stage B2	Stage C1	Stage C2	Stage D
Disease progression	Tumor is restricted to the mucosa only	Tumor invades into the muscularis propria	Tumor invades through the muscularis propria and serosa	Tumor invades the muscularis propria and is found in regional lymph nodes	Tumor invades the muscularis propria (and extends into the serosa) and is found in regional lymph nodes	Tumor has metastasized to distant organs such as liver, lungs, and bone
Estimated 5-year survival	90%	80%	60%	40%	40%	< 5%

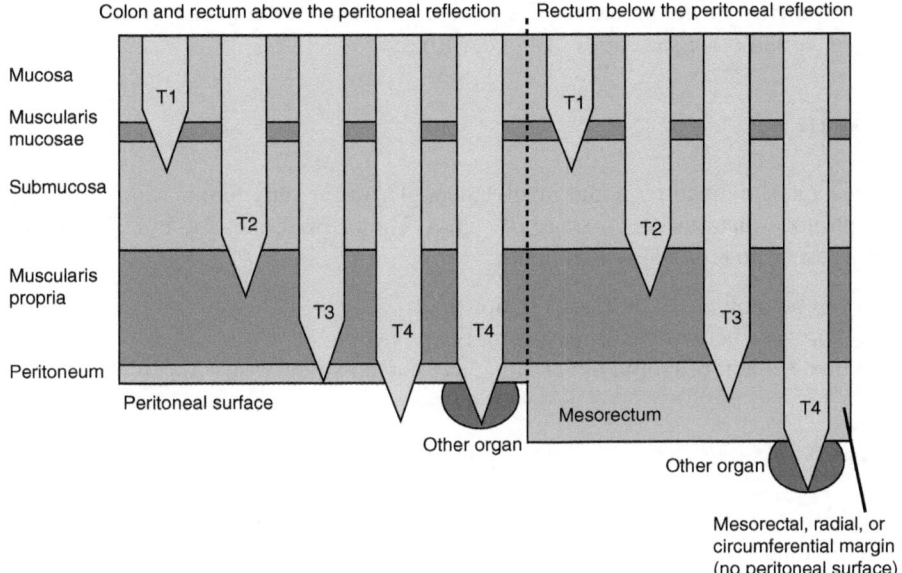

Fig. 5.10 TNM staging of colorectal cancer

TNM Classification

The American Joint Committee for cancer staging and end results developed this system as an alternative to the Dukes' classification system. The TNM system (T: tumor; N: nodes; M: metastases) analyzes in detail the degree of local and regional spread of the tumor (see Fig. 5.10).

Stage 0

Carcinoma in situ.

Stage I

Tumor extends into the submucosa (T1, N0, M0).
Tumor extends to and invades the muscularis propria (T2, N0, M0).

Stage II

Tumor extends to and invades the subserosa, nonperitonealized pericolonic tissue, or perirectal tissue (T3, N0, M0).

Tumor extends to and perforates the visceral peritoneum or directly invades nearby organs and other structures (T4, N0, M0).

Stage III

This stage is defined by nodal involvement. Therefore, any tumor with associated lymph node metastasis is a stage III tumor. Tumor perforates the bowel wall and metastasizes to regional lymph nodes.

N1: 1–3 pericolonic or perirectal lymph nodes.
N2: 4 or more pericolonic or perirectal lymph nodes.
N3: Involvement of lymph nodes along any named vascular structure.

Stage IV

Tumor has metastasized to distant organs such as the liver, lungs, and bone. Microscopic grading of the degree of differentiation of the tumor is also used to determine prognosis. Pathologic grading is as follows:

Grade 1 (well differentiated) —epithelial proliferation.
Grade 2 (moderately differentiated) —glandular pattern present but more crowded.
Grade 3 (poorly differentiated) —anaplastic cells, frequent mitosis.
Grade 4 (mucinous tumors) —more than 50% of tumor volume is occupied by mucin.

Surgery for Rectal Cancer (See Chaps. 18–21)

General Information

Several different surgical techniques are employed for rectal cancer depending on the location and the tumor stage. The primary goal of surgery is the complete removal of the tumor. When possible, surgical techniques are also employed that result in the preservation of continence. Recent advances in surgical therapy, particularly with the improvement of low anterior resections with double-stapling devices, have allowed more patients to avoid the requirement of a permanent ostomy after surgery for rectal cancer (see Chap. 20).

Abdominoperineal Resection (APR)

APR is performed when there is an inadequate distal margin of the rectum (<2 cm); when there is a large, bulky pelvic tumor present; and when there is evidence of local tumor extension beyond the rectum (see Chap. 21). This surgery involves an

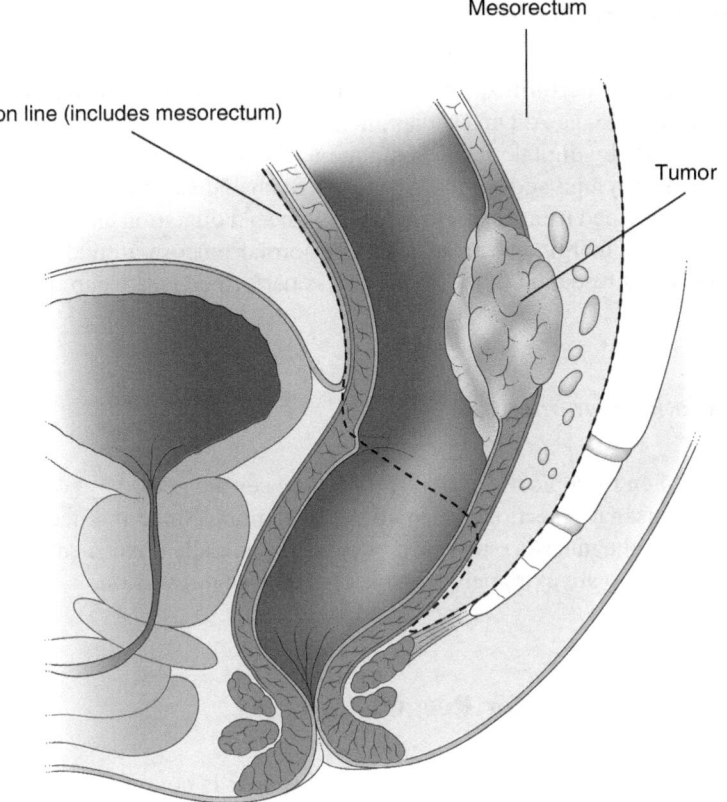

Fig. 5.11   The area removed during mesorectal resection

en bloc dissection of the retroperitoneum between the ureters, resulting in removal of the anus, rectum, and distal sigmoid colon. Complete removal of the rectal mesentery (mesorectum) with lymph node removal (total mesorectal excision) is also usually performed (see Fig. 5.11). A permanent sigmoid colostomy is constructed.

Low Anterior Resection

This surgery is performed when there is at least a 2-cm margin of normal tissue distal to the tumor. The development of the double stapling technique has allowed an increased number of patients with more distal rectal tumors to undergo low anterior resections and avoid an APR (see Chap. 21). Coloanal anastomosis and the occasional construction of colonic J pouches are also new surgical techniques allowing preservation of the anal sphincters and avoidance of APR. Complete mesorectal excision has also been advocated in conjunction with low anterior resections and has been repeatedly demonstrated to reduce the local recurrence rate of rectal cancers (see Chap. 18).

Transanal Resection

This surgery is performed on tumors that are ≤4 cm in diameter and involve the mucosa only (Stage A, Dukes' classification). These tumors should be palpable and freely mobile by digital rectal examination. Tumors should be <9 cm from the anal verge and no lymph nodes should be detected on endoscopic ultrasound. The procedure is performed using a proctoscope or with anal dilatation and retractor insertion. Removal of a margin (of about 1 cm) of normal mucosa around the tumor with a full-thickness resection of the rectal wall is performed (see Chap. 19).

Additional Comments

The use of endoscopic mucosal resection has been advocated by some as an alternative to transanal resection for small rectal tumors. Since this technique involves resection of the mucosa only this procedure is generally advocated for rectal cancer in patients who are extremely high-risk for transanal resection.

Medical Therapy for Rectal Cancer

Local recurrence after resection for rectal cancer is common (average 30% local recurrence rate). Patients with TNM stage II (Dukes' B2) rectal cancer have a 25–30% likelihood of local recurrence and those with TNM stage III (Dukes' C) have a >50% probability of local recurrence. Local recurrence in patients with TNM stage I appears to be less than 10%. Pre- or postoperative radiation therapy significantly reduces the rate of local recurrence but does not appear to significantly affect long-term survival. Recent studies have demonstrated that postoperative combination radiation therapy and chemotherapy significantly improve patient survival and reduce both local and systemic postoperative recurrences in patients with TNM stage II (Dukes' B2) and TNM stage III (Dukes' C) rectal cancer.

Current Therapy for TNM Stage II and III Rectal Cancer

Pre- or postoperative radiation therapy combined with 5-fluorouracil (5-FU) and leucovorin, or 5-FU and levamisole is used. Adjuvant chemotherapy is usually well tolerated. This regimen is also used for metastatic disease, resulting in mild improvement in survival and quality of life.

Side Effects of 5-FU

Common

Dermatitis, alopecia, stomatitis, nausea, vomiting, diarrhea, anorexia, and mucositis.

Serious

Myelosuppression, hypotension, coronary ischemia, gastrointestinal ulceration, hepatitis, coagulopathy, and dyspnea.

Side Effects of Levamisole

Common

Nausea, vomiting, diarrhea, constipation, dermatitis, alopecia, fatigue, fever, arthralgia, and myalgia.

Serious

Acute neurologic toxicity, myelosuppression, secondary infection, and depression.

Side Effects of Leucovorin

Rare cases of allergic or anaphylactoid reactions have been reported.

Side Effects of Radiation Therapy

Acute

Diarrhea, rectal pain, urgency, and urinary frequency.

Chronic

Rectal bleeding, fecal incontinence, urgency, rectal pain, and diarrhea.

Other Rectal Malignancies

Carcinoid Tumor

Epidemiology

Carcinoid tumors are rare and occur in less than 0.001% of the general population. Only 12% originate in the rectum. The average age of presentation of rectal carcinoid tumors is 58 years, and they are equally common in men and women. Carcinoid tumors are seen in up to 10% of individuals with multiple endocrine neoplasia (MEN) syndromes.

Pathophysiology

Carcinoid tumors arise from neuroendocrine cells of ectodermal origin. These cells are able to secrete a variety of hormones and other biologically active compounds. The tumors usually appear as small rectal nodules and are often found incidentally when small polyps are removed during routine colonoscopy.

Symptoms

Carcinoid tumors are most often asymptomatic. However, symptoms such as rectal bleeding or rectal pain may be present. Advanced stage tumors may cause symptoms such as weight loss and anorexia.

Diagnostic Testing

Digital rectal examination may reveal a palpable nodule. Endoscopic evaluation and biopsy are required for diagnosis (see Fig. 5.12).

Treatment

Endoscopic small lesions (<1 cm) can be removed in their entirety by endoscopy. Transanal resection may be performed for lesions <2 cm in diameter. Larger lesions are treated by rectal resection with anastomosis or APR (see Chap. 21).

Prognosis

Complete resection of lesions results in resolution of the disease. Lesions that are >2 cm in diameter have a high likelihood of metastasis (>60%), and patients may have carcinoid tumors in other portions of the bowel. Five-year survival is approximately 75% for all rectal carcinoid tumors.

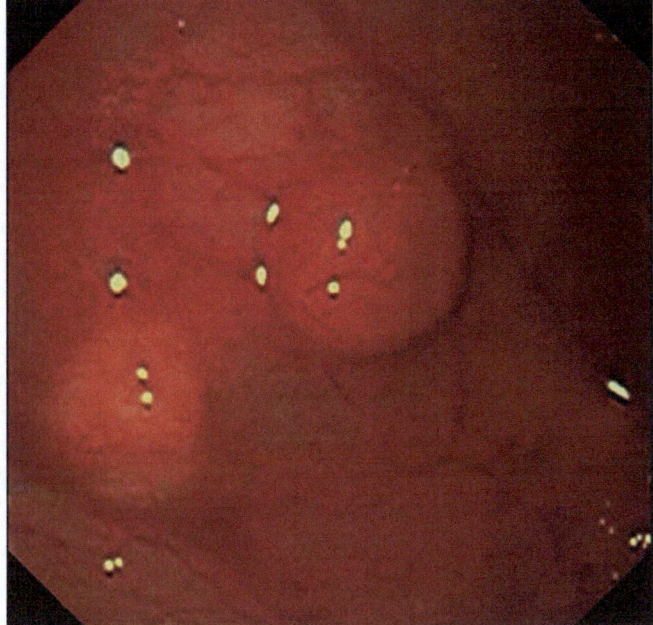

Fig. 5.12 Polypoid colonic lesion without specific endoscopic appearances found to be a carcinoid tumor on histologic evaluation

Leiomyosarcoma

Epidemiology

This is a rare colonic tumor that most often occurs in the rectum.

Pathophysiology

Leiomyosarcoma is a slow-growing tumor that originates from intestinal smooth muscle cells. Local extension into perirectal tissue is a common finding.

Symptoms

The most common symptoms are rectal pain and bleeding.

Diagnosis

It is usually possible to detect the tumors on digital rectal examination. Endoscopy and biopsy are utilized to make the diagnosis.

Treatment

Rectal resection is the treatment of choice (see Chap. 21).

Prognosis

The predicted 5-year survival rate after diagnosis of rectal leiomyosarcoma is 20%.

Lymphoma

Epidemiology

Primary rectal lymphoma is very rare (<0.1% of all malignant rectal neoplasms). Colonic lymphoma occurs most frequently in the cecum.

Risk Factors

Immunodeficiency syndromes, HIV infection, and, possibly, treatment with immunosuppressive agents.

Treatment

Resection of the tumor alone or in combination with radiation therapy is used for primary intestinal lymphoma if there is no evidence of disease beyond the rectum (see Chap. 21). Otherwise, tumor staging followed by resection, chemotherapy, and/ or radiation therapy may be utilized.

Metastatic Rectal Tumors

Definition

Metastatic rectal tumors are tumors that may metastasize or extend to the rectum. These tumors may metastasize locally from the prostate or uterus, or further afield from the ovaries, kidneys, pancreas, duodenum, stomach, breast, or lung.

Symptoms

The main symptoms are rectal bleeding, rectal pain, and obstruction.

Diagnosis

Digital rectal examination, endoscopy, and biopsy are utilized to make the diagnosis.

Treatment

Usually palliative with fecal diversion if obstructive symptoms are present. Resection is reserved for intractable bleeding.

Chapter 6
Infectious Disorders of the Anus and Rectum

Eli D. Ehrenpreis

Chlamydia and Lymphogranuloma Venereum

Organism

Chlamydia trachomatis. Twelve serologic variants (serovars) have been identified. Serovars D–K cause sexually transmitted urethritis and anorectal infections, and serovars L1–L3 cause lymphogranuloma venereum (LGV).

Epidemiology

C. trachomatis infection is the most common sexually transmitted disease in the United States, and LGV is 20 times more common in men than in women.

Patients at Risk

Homosexual males, African-Americans, patients infected with HIV, and other individuals at risk of contracting venereal diseases, for example, people with multiple sex partners or who are immunocompromised.

E.D. Ehrenpreis, MD (✉)
Chief of Gastroenterology and Endoscopy, Highland Park Hospital,
NorthShore University Health System, Highland Park, IL 60035, USA

Clinical Associate Professor of Medicine, University of Chicago Medical Center,
Highland Park, IL 60035, USA
e-mail: ehrenpreis@gipharm.net

E.D. Ehrenpreis et al. (eds.), *Anal and Rectal Diseases: A Concise Manual*,
DOI 10.1007/978-1-4614-1102-4_6, © Springer Science+Business Media, LLC 2012

Mode of Transmission

Sexually transmitted.

Incubation Time

Clinical course. Several forms of *C. trachomatis* infection occur. Genital tract infection in males or females may be asymptomatic or result in the development of urethral discharge and/or dysuria, or ascending infections such as salpingitis. In males with LGV, a shallow ulcer first appears on the penis. Marked inguinal adenopathy (buboes) with fever, chills, and headache follows. Late stages of the disease are characterized by rectal or colorectal involvement (proctitis and colitis), rectal strictures, and rectovaginal fistulas. Proctocolitis may occur as the initial presentation in a severe form of the disease seen in homosexual males.

Pathophysiology

Extensive inflammation results in diffuse infiltration, abscesses, and granuloma formation. Ulceration of the mucosa is seen on endoscopy.

Diagnostic Testing

Flexible sigmoidoscopy, biopsies, rectal culture, and microimmunofluorescent antibody or complement fixation testing.

Treatment

The treatments for *C. trachomatis* infection are shown in Table 6.1.

Clinical Pearls

Patients should be empirically treated for gonococcal proctitis if they are diagnosed with chlamydial proctitis. Sexual partners should also undergo treatment.

Table 6.1 Treatments and their course for patients with *C. trachomatis* infection

Treatment	Course
Azithromycin	Single dose of 1 g for 7 days
Doxycycline	100 mg b.i.d. for 7 days
Tetracycline	500 mg q.i.d. for 21 days
Erythromycin	500 mg q.i.d. for 21 days
Trimethoprim–sulfamethoxazole	Double strength b.i.d. for 21 days

Gonorrhea

Organism

Neisseria gonorrhoeae, a Gram-negative, intracellular diplococcus.

Epidemiology

From 400,000 to 800,000 cases of gonorrhea occur annually in the United States. There is an incidence of infection of 5% in high-risk groups at any given time.

Patients at Risk

Homosexual males, particularly those practicing receptive anal intercourse; women with pelvic inflammatory disease; and males and females with other sexually transmitted diseases.

Mode of Transmission

Sexual intercourse, receptive anal intercourse, or spread from genital infection.

Incubation Time

Symptoms begin 5–7 days after exposure.

Symptoms

Typical

Diarrhea, mucopurulent discharge, and urgency.

Additional

Arthritis, tenosynovitis, and skin rash.

Pathophysiology

Infection causes inflammation of the rectum characterized by mucosal erosions, erythema, and friability.

Diagnostic Tests

Rectal swab or biopsy testing with Gram stain and culture using Thayer–Martin medium (see Fig. 6.1).

Treatment

The standard treatment is a single 250-mg dose of ceftriaxone administered intramuscularly. Patients should also receive treatment for possible concomitant chlamydial infection with, for example, 100 mg doxycycline b.i.d. for 21 days.

Clinical Pearls

Repeated cultures may be necessary due to difficulty in culturing *N. gonorrhoeae*. This condition is extremely common in homosexual males visiting sexually transmitted disease clinics.

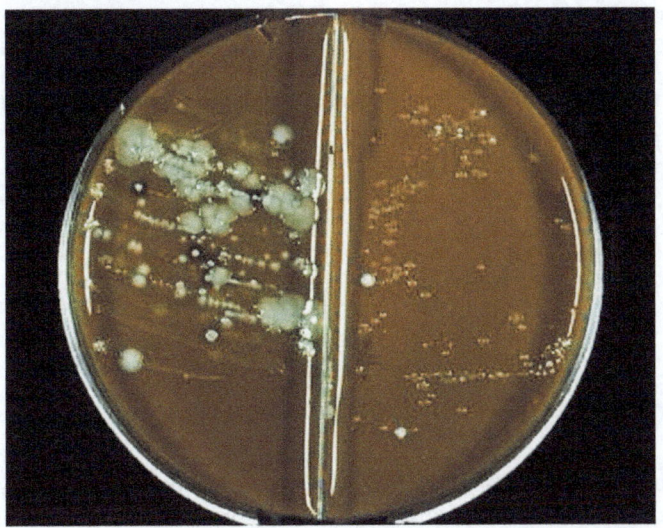

Fig. 6.1 A Thayer–Martin bi-plane culture for *N. gonorrhoeae*. The *left side* of the plane is chocolate agar; the *right side* contains chocolate agar plus antibiotics, which block growth of normal flora and allow the gonococcus to grow

Herpes Simplex

Organism

Herpes simplex virus 2 (HSV-2).

Epidemiology

Unlike human papilloma virus exposure, which commonly results in infection, perianal and rectal infection with herpes simplex is rare.

Patients at Risk

Homosexual males practicing receptive anal intercourse, people with multiple sex partners, and prior history of genital herpes infection.

Mode of Transmission

Sexual or anal intercourse: It may be spread from the mouth or genital tract.

Incubation Time

From 2 to 7 days. It may be delayed by up to 3 weeks.

Symptoms

Severe pain with defecation, tenesmus, diarrhea, mucopurulent discharge from rectum, and pruritus ani. Marked discomfort occurs with digital rectal examination or sigmoidoscopy.

Pathophysiology

Initial symptoms may appear within a few days of exposure and include pruritus ani or paresthesia. Subsequently, vesicles form in the perianal region and rectum. Mucosal friability, ulcerations, and pustules may follow.

Diagnostic Testing

Sigmoidoscopy (usually performed with anesthesia because of discomfort) and/or scrapings or biopsies of anorectal ulcers for viral culture. Multinucleated giant cells with classic intranuclear inclusion bodies are seen on light microscopy.

Treatment

The standard treatment is 400 mg oral acyclovir 5 times daily. Foscarnet is used for resistant cases.

Clinical Pearls

Biopsies or scrapings must be obtained from the edge of the ulcers, since organisms are not present in necrotic tissue and exudates in the central portion of the ulcers. Oral maintenance therapy with acyclovir is often used to suppress further herpes outbreaks.

HIV-Associated Anorectal Disease

Epidemiology

Anorectal disorders have been described in 6–33% of HIV-infected patients, and symptoms of anorectal disease are the most common indication (85%) for referral to surgery in this patient group. Approximately 50% of HIV-infected patients with anorectal disorders will require surgery.

Patients at Risk

High-risk groups for HIV infection include homosexual males and intravenous drug abusers. The incidence of sexually transmitted HIV has been increasing in the heterosexual population. Anorectal complications occur in the majority of HIV-infected homosexual males but are uncommon in HIV-positive intravenous drug abusers. Advanced HIV infection has been associated with the development of complex anal abscesses, chronic anal ulcers, and severe perianal sepsis. Anal malignancies associated with HIV occur almost exclusively in homosexual males.

Symptoms

Symptoms vary according to individual conditions (see individual chapters for complete descriptions, including infectious conditions, neoplasms of the anus, anorectal abscess, perianal fistula, anal fissure, hemorrhoids, and diarrhea). Fecal incontinence in the absence of significant anorectal pathology may be seen in patients with late-stage HIV infection as a result of severe diarrhea. Kaposi's sarcoma and non-Hodgkin's lymphoma generally present with pain, abscesses, or anorectal bleeding.

Pathophysiology

Anorectal disorders in HIV-infected patients can be classified as follows:

1. Common anorectal pathology
2. Condylomata acuminata (venereal warts)
3. Perianal sepsis (including fistulas and abscesses)
4. Anorectal ulcerations
5. Anorectal malignancies (Kaposi's sarcoma, non-Hodgkin's lymphoma, and squamous cell carcinoma of the anal canal or anal margin).

Immunodeficiency often modifies the presentation of these diseases. For example, the development of anal abscesses in patients with advanced HIV infection may be associated with severe septic complications including necrotizing gangrene and "metastatic abscesses" in the liver, brain, and mediastinum. HIV infection is a definitive risk factor for the development of carcinoma in situ or invasive squamous cell carcinoma from anal or genital condylomata. Ulceration of the anal canal and perianal region is a unique manifestation of HIV infection.

Diagnostic Testing

Physical examination, flexible sigmoidoscopy with biopsy, and/or examination under anesthesia with biopsy.

Treatment/Clinical Pearls

Treatments vary according to the condition. Anal abscesses are treated aggressively to prevent septic complications. Conservative management is suggested for anal fissures seen in patients with advanced HIV infection due to the risk of fecal incontinence and poor wound healing associated with surgical management. Hemorrhoids are also managed conservatively: rubber band ligation is to be avoided as cases of Fournier's gangrene (localized necrosis of the scrotum) have complicated this procedure in immunocompromised patients. Fournier's gangrene develops when anaerobic organisms enter potential spaces in the groin following an initial infection at the banding site. Anal condylomata should be managed by surgical excision or fulguration instead of medical therapy due to the high-risk for the development of anorectal neoplasms in partially treated lesions. Avoidance of receptive anal intercourse is suggested in patients with HIV-associated anal ulcerations. Intralesional steroids have been used for this condition. In general, conservative management of these conditions is recommended because of the risk of surgical complications and decreased wound healing in late-stage HIV infection.

Syphilis

Organism

Treponema pallidum.

Epidemiology

The incidence of *T. pallidum* infection is increasing. Currently, 20 cases are seen per 100,000 people in the United States. The organism is highly contagious; 30–50% of sexual partners of people infected with syphilis contract the disease.

Patients at Risk

Homosexual males practicing receptive anal intercourse and people with multiple sexual partners.

Mode of Transmission

Sexually transmitted.

Incubation Time

Two to eight weeks.

Symptoms

May be relatively asymptomatic or produce severe anorectal discomfort, purulent anal discharge, difficulty with rectal evacuation, and tenesmus.

Pathophysiology

The initial lesion is termed a "chancre" (primary syphilis), a well-demarcated ulcer that begins at the site of infection. This progresses to disseminated anorectal disease characterized by ulceration, fissuring, fistulas, proctitis, and lymphadenopathy. A reddish rash due to systemic infection (secondary syphilis) follows after 2–10 weeks.

Diagnostic Testing

Anorectal swab with dark-field examination, serologic testing, and/or immunofluorescent staining.

Treatment

Benzathine penicillin 2.4 million units intramuscularly repeated after 7 days. Tetracycline (500 mg q.i.d. for 15 days) or erythromycin (500 mg q.i.d. for 30 days) is given to patients who are allergic to penicillin.

Clinical Pearls

Because this is a difficult infection to diagnose, patients with risk factors who are suspected of having anorectal syphilis should be treated empirically.

Venereal Warts (Condylomata Acuminata)

Organism

Human papilloma DNA virus (HPV) from the papovavirus family. At least 60 subtypes of HPV have been identified. Of these subtypes, 6, 11, 16, 18, 31, 33, 35, 45, 51, 52, and 56 are sexually transmitted. Subtypes 16 and 18 are consistently associated with the development of cervical cancer.

Epidemiology

HPV is the most common sexually transmitted viral infection. The incidence of condylomata acuminata is approximately one million cases per year in the United States. The condition is highly contagious; up to 70% of the sexual partners of those infected will contract the disease.

Patients at Risk

Sexual partners of infected individuals; sexually promiscuous people; homosexual males; patients with other sexually transmitted diseases such as gonorrhea, syphilis, and genital herpes; and victims of childhood sexual abuse.

Mode of Transmission

Sexual. All sexually transmitted subtypes are associated with the development of anogenital warts.

Incubation Time

Warts appear within 3–4 months of exposure to the virus.

Symptoms

Fullness or a mass-like sensation in the perianal or genital region, pruritus ani, perianal or genital pain, rectal bleeding, and discharge.

Pathophysiology

Anal infection causes squamous cell proliferation with multiple papillomas developing in the anal canal and urogenital area. Squamous metaplasia may occur with long-standing infection, particularly with HPV subtypes 16 and 18. After a number of years, carcinoma in situ with progression to invasive squamous cell carcinoma may develop with infections of subtypes 16 or 18.

Diagnostic Testing

Physical examination reveals characteristic findings: single or multiple warts with a cauliflower-like appearance are seen in the affected area (see Fig. 6.2). The anal canal is affected in up to 90% of patients, and lesions frequently extend proximally to the dentate line. Biopsies show squamous cell proliferation and loss of the keratinized layer of the skin (acanthosis and hyperkeratosis). Proctoscopy or flexible sigmoidoscopy is required to determine the extent of anal and rectal involvement.

Treatment

Topical Therapy with Destructive Antiviral Agents

Destruction of venereal warts with 25% podophyllin (a cytotoxic agent) in tincture of benzoin is a commonly performed, office-based procedure. After thorough cleansing, a small quantity is applied directly to the lesions (by a physician only).

Fig. 6.2 Physical examination shows cauliflower-like appearance of lesions

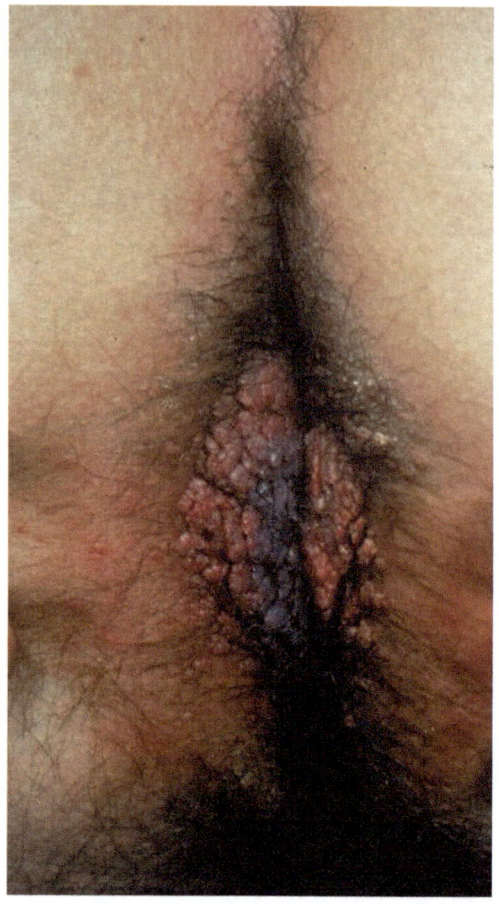

The solution is left in contact with the wart for 30 min during the first session and for 1–4 h during follow-up treatments, which are conducted weekly until either the warts are destroyed or the patient develops intolerance to treatment. The solution is removed from the area by cleansing with soap and water. The goal of the treatment is to completely destroy the warts. Physicians must be cautious when applying the tincture since application to large areas increases the risk of systemic absorption and toxicity.

Podofilox is an antimitotic agent, which is available in a 0.5% gel or topical solution. Podofilox can be applied to the affected area by the patient and is usually with a cotton tip applicator. The patient should apply podofilox twice daily for 3 days and stop treatment for 4 days, resuming treatment on day 8. This weekly cycle is continued until complete elimination of warts has been achieved. In clinical trials, approximately 50% of patients achieved complete clearance of lesions after 2–4 weeks of treatment.

Imiquimod (Aldara) is an agent that promotes cytokine action, thus increasing local antiviral immune activity. It is applied to the affected area three times per week and left in place for 6–10 h. These treatments are continued until warts are cleared, or for up to 16 weeks. Treated areas may also be covered with nonocclusive dressings. Imiquimod has been demonstrated to be effective in more than 50% of patients using the medication.

Other Topical Treatments

Cryotherapy, laser therapy, electrocoagulative therapy, and injection of interferon and other cytotoxic agents into lesions.

Surgical

Surgery is recommended for larger clusters of lesions, intrarectal lesions, refractory lesions, and recurrent lesions. Local anesthetic and epinephrine are injected into the base of the lesion(s) prior to removal with surgical scissors and forceps.

Clinical Pearls

Patients with smaller lesions and less extensive involvement are usually treated with the topical destructive agents podophyllin or podofilox. Patients who do not respond to these therapies (10–50%) are referred for other forms of topical therapy or surgery. Some authors have suggested periodic surveillance for anal and genital cancer in affected individuals. Recurrence of symptoms should prompt immediate evaluation of the previously treated area. Recurrence of genital warts is a common phenomenon. Women with condylomata acuminata should undergo regular Pap smears since they are at high risk for the development of cervical dysplasia and carcinoma.

Chapter 7
Miscellaneous Anorectal Conditions

Eli D. Ehrenpreis

Diarrhea

Epidemiology

Self-limited diarrhea is extremely common. The passage of loose or watery stools without abdominal pain was found to occur in 4.3% of males and 2.2% of females surveyed in Bristol, UK during a 1-year period. Chronic diarrhea is thought to affect 5% of the adult population annually in the United States, and approximately 450,000 patients are hospitalized.

Patients at Risk

People with diabetes, celiac sprue, pancreatic disorders, or small intestinal disorders; travelers to Third World countries; HIV-infected patients; people on antibiotics; patients undergoing or having had radiation therapy; patients who have had surgery of the stomach, small intestine, or colon; and individuals receiving enteric formula feedings. A variety of medications and herbal preparations have laxative effects.

E.D. Ehrenpreis, MD (✉)
Chief of Gastroenterology and Endoscopy, Highland Park Hospital,
NorthShore University Health System, Highland Park, IL 60035, USA

Clinical Associate Professor of Medicine, University of Chicago Medical Center,
Highland Park, IL 60035, USA
e-mail: ehrenpreis@gipharm.net

E.D. Ehrenpreis et al. (eds.), *Anal and Rectal Diseases: A Concise Manual*,
DOI 10.1007/978-1-4614-1102-4_7, © Springer Science+Business Media, LLC 2012

Pathophysiology

Diarrhea occurs when the normal absorptive mechanism of the small intestine and colon is overwhelmed by excessive fluid secretion and hypermotility. The overall result is the passage of multiple frequent stools. Diarrhea is most objectively defined as the passage of more than 200 mL (200 g) of stool per day. Diarrhea can be divided into several categories, which are outlined in the following sections, together with common causes of each.

Acute

Symptoms lasting from several days to 4 weeks. The majority of cases of acute diarrhea are due to viral, bacterial, or parasitic infection.

Chronic

Symptoms lasting >4 weeks. A large number of conditions can result in the development of chronic diarrhea. Chronic diarrhea may be further divided into two main categories: osmotic diarrhea and secretory diarrhea (See Chapter 2 Quantitative Stool Collection).

Osmotic Diarrhea

Malabsorbed or poorly absorbed sugars, other carbohydrates, and other osmotically active substances (such as magnesium) produce laxative effects by inducing the secretion of water. Since the overall osmolality of stool must remain at approximately 290 mOsm/L, the presence of osmotically active substances in the colonic lumen results in net water secretion and increased stool volume.

Secretory Diarrhea

A variety of conditions – including hypermotility, infectious and inflammatory disorders, excessive secretion of chloride or bicarbonate, or decreased absorption of sodium – result in release of fluids and electrolytes.

Symptoms

Passage of frequent watery or soft stools. Severe diarrhea may be associated with dehydration and consequent electrolyte disturbance. Frequent small stools with cramping and urgency suggest proctitis or left-sided colitis (see Fig. 7.1). Large volume stools suggest a small intestinal source of diarrhea. Bloating, flatulence, and foul smelling and oily stools occur in malabsorptive states. Recent foreign travel suggests the presence of an infectious source.

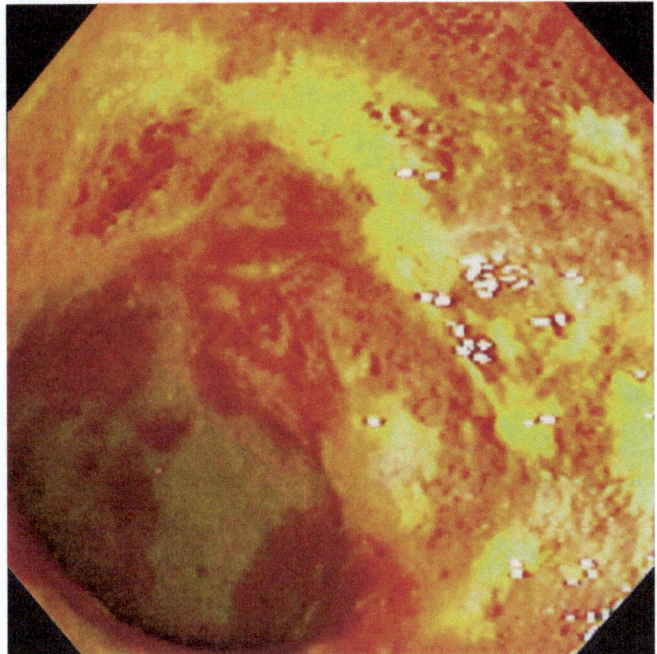

Fig. 7.1 Infectious colitis due to cytomegalovirus in a patient with chronic myelogenous leukemia

Diagnostic Testing

A stool sample should be obtained, checked for parasites and *Clostridium difficile* toxin, and cultured. Other evaluations include fecal volume, fecal fat, electrolyte and pH measurement, complete blood count, serum chemistries, celiac sprue panel, thyroid-stimulating hormone, flexible sigmoidoscopy, colonoscopy, small intestine biopsy, and 24-h urine test for 5-hydroxyindole acetic acid (5-HIAA).

Treatment

Identification of the underlying source of this symptom is critical for initiating proper therapy. It is best to control diarrhea by direct treatment of the cause. Treatments may include anti-inflammatory agents for inflammatory bowel disease and a gluten-free diet for celiac sprue. Treatments that may provide relief of the symptoms of diarrhea in the presence or absence of organic disorders include fiber, opioids, cholestyramine, octreotide, and anticholinergic agents.

Clinical Pearls

A careful history will assist in differentiating various causes of diarrhea. The possibility of laxative abuse should not be ignored. Patients with diarrhea and fecal incontinence generally experience improvement in their symptoms of incontinence when their diarrhea is under control.

Fecal Impaction

Definition

Fecal impaction is the development of a colonic obstruction due to filling of the lumen with a large, hard stool. It occurs most commonly in the rectum.

Epidemiology

The rising incidence of fecal impaction parallels the increasing prevalence of chronic constipation. Fecal impaction is the cause of colonic obstruction in up to 50% of bedridden patients in nursing homes and patients with spinal cord injuries.

Patients at Risk

Patients with spinal cord injuries and bedridden patients are at high risk. Constipation may occur in up to 25% of the elderly population and is three times more common in women than in men. A variety of medications – including calcium channel blockers, anticholinergics, opioids, antidepressants, and antipsychotics – predispose to constipation and, therefore, the development of fecal impaction. A number of neurologic diseases (Parkinson's disease, dementia, multiple sclerosis) are associated with decreased colonic function and constipation, therefore placing patients at risk for fecal impaction. Endocrine disorders including diabetes and hypothyroidism are additional risk factors. Dehydration increases the likelihood of developing fecal impaction in high-risk patients.

Symptoms

Constipation, rectal pain, and a sensation of a rectal mass are common symptoms. Other symptoms, including diarrhea and fecal incontinence due to overflow of liquid stool past the impacted fecal bolus, may be present. Patients with neurologic diseases or spinal cord injury may be unaware of the presence of the fecal impaction. In addition, fecal impaction in patients with spinal cord injury may lead to autonomic dysreflexia, a medical emergency characterized by the acute development of symptomatic hypertension with hyperactive reflexes. Rectal bleeding may occur in patients with stercoral ulcers (see Section "Pathophysiology"). In extreme cases of fecal impaction, colonic obstruction with abdominal distention and signs and symptoms of bowel perforation or peritonitis may be present.

Pathophysiology

Decreased neuromuscular function of the colon results in colonic hypomotility, prolonged transit time in the colon, and fecal retention. Increased contact time between fecal material and the colon results in firm, dehydrated stools. A vicious cycle may develop in which increasing stool retention further delays motility and produces even drier, firmer stools. Altered sensorium may exacerbate the problem through the loss of normal impulses to defecate. A hard stool may be retained for such a prolonged period of time in a single segment of the colon that ischemic ulceration – a stercoral ulcer – may occur.

Diagnostic Testing

Examination of the abdomen may reveal the presence of soft or firm masses, particularly over the left colon. Digital rectal examination will reveal a firm, mobile mass in the rectum. An abdominal X-ray will demonstrate the presence of stool accumulation in the colon. A sigmoidoscopy may be required to rule out other types of rectal mass, for example, carcinoma.

Treatment

Most forms of fecal impaction can be treated with digital fecal disimpaction. However, this procedure may produce marked discomfort and even hypotension in some patients, and, therefore, some form of sedation should be considered. Following the removal of the largest and most obstructive fecal boluses, follow-up with gentle enema therapy is performed. In patients who have developed fecal impaction, a bowel regimen including laxatives and enemas on a regular basis is suggested.

Clinical Pearls

It is particularly important to remind patients who are on medications that cause constipation to consume large volumes of liquid on a daily basis, for example five to eight glasses of water or other nonalcoholic fluids daily. Patients who have an episode of fecal impaction should be placed on a regular regimen of stool softeners and/or osmotic laxatives as a prophylaxis against further episodes.

Pilonidal Sinuses

Epidemiology

Symptomatic pilonidal sinuses generally develop between the ages of 20 and 30 years. Three-quarters of cases are seen in males. There is some suggestion that trauma to the skin overlying the sacrococcygeal region (such as strenuous activity and sitting in vehicles in rugged environments – as seen in military personnel) may increase the likelihood of development of the condition.

Symptoms

If an abscess is present, pain may be the predominant symptom. Otherwise, patients will notice swelling, drainage, and tenderness of the affected area.

Pathophysiology

Pilonidal sinuses develop in the intergluteal cleft and in the skin overlying the sacrum and coccygeal bone (see Fig. 7.2). The condition develops when a sinus

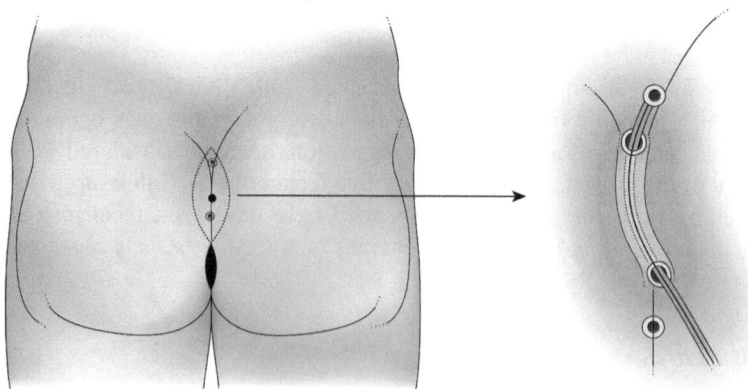

Fig. 7.2 Pilonidal sinus. On examination, pits or external openings in the intergluteal cleft are seen. The openings often communicate with each other, as shown on the *right*

tract forms following an episode of folliculitis and abscess formation. The initiating factor may be a plug of keratin that develops in the hair follicle. Shafts of hair entering a previously developed sinus may also initiate the condition. Recurrent abscesses, infection, and multiple sinus tracts may be seen.

Diagnosis

Physical examination reveals an area of inflammation, tenderness, and erythema in the gluteal crease, usually 5–7 cm from the anal opening. Hair follicles will often be noted at the site of the lesion, and there is often more than one sinus opening. The presence of hair follicles and the lack of an opening from within the anorectal region differentiate pilonidal cysts from anal and rectal fistulas.

Treatment

If an abscess is present, incision and drainage are the treatments of choice, followed by complete excision when the acute process is resolved. Shaving hair from the intergluteal cleft on a weekly basis decreases the chance of recurrence.

Clinical Pearls

Recurrences following excision of the pilonidal sinus need additional excisions. In refractory cases, more extensive excision surgery may be required.

Rectal Foreign Bodies

Epidemiology

The majority of the foreign bodies found in the rectum have been placed there rectally; however, swallowed objects may occasionally lodge in the rectum. Foreign bodies may be introduced either intentionally (autoeroticism, sexual activity, rape) or unintentionally (as a means of dislodging impacted stool).

Patients at Risk

Homosexuals, individuals practicing receptive anal sex utilizing foreign objects, rape victims, children, people with altered sensorium, and patients with rectal or anal strictures (in the case of swallowed objects).

Pathophysiology

After placing large objects in the rectum, intense anal spasm and/or pain sometimes prevent simple removal. A sharp swallowed object may lodge itself in normal rectal mucosa. Other swallowed objects may become impacted at the rectosigmoid junction. Narrowed luminal caliber secondary to strictures or diverticular disease increases the likelihood of impaction.

Symptoms

Pain in the abdomen or rectum, rectal bleeding, discharge, and symptoms of peritonitis (abdominal distention, fever, peritoneal signs).

Diagnostic Testing

Physical examination should include careful abdominal examination to rule out peritonitis. The abdomen should be palpated for masses and the anus should be carefully inspected for evidence of fissure and/or anal trauma. Prior to the performance of a rectal examination, an abdominal X-ray should be performed. Subsequently, a digital rectal exam can be carefully performed (as long as a sharp object is not suspected). Assessment of anal sphincter tone is recommended. Patients may require anesthesia for adequate examination.

Treatment

Following adequate anesthesia, small objects may be digitally removed. Endoscopic removal may be possible in selected cases; removal of sharp objects requires an overtube. General anesthesia is used for the removal of larger objects. This can be performed using a variety of devices including obstetric forceps and modified padded pliers. After the insertion of a rigid proctoscope, a Foley catheter or a

Sengstaken–Blakemore tube may be inflated proximal to the object, which is then pulled down toward the anus. Patients who have evidence of peritonitis will require laparotomy (see Chap. 23).

Clinical Pearls

The rectosigmoid region should be visualized endoscopically following removal of a foreign object to ensure that it has been completely removed and to rule out mucosal injury.

Part II
Surgical

Chapter 8
Surgery for Anal Fissure

Marc Singer and Shmuel Avital

Description of Procedure

Treatment of an anal fissure, either medical or surgical, is aimed at relaxation of the hypertonic internal sphincter. Breaking the cycle of spasm of the sphincter will allow for healing of the fissure. Lateral internal sphincterotomy is the primary surgical procedure used to treat anal fissure.

Indications

Patients who have failed a course of medical management including topical muscle relaxants (nitroglycerin, nifedipine, or diltiazem) and/or botulinum toxin injections are eligible candidates for sphincterotomy. Alternatively, patients desiring more immediate relief of symptoms are potential surgical candidates.

Contraindications

The primary contraindication of sphincterotomy is preexisting fecal incontinence. The operation divides sphincter muscle, and patients with previous issues with incontinence may experience worsening postoperative control of stool.

M. Singer, MD (✉)
Department of Surgery, Division of Colon and Rectal Surgery, NorthShore University Health System, 2650 Ridge Avenue, Ste 2507, Evanston, IL 60201, USA
e-mail: msinger1@northshore.org

S. Avital, MD
Chief of Surgery, Department of Surgery B, Meir Medical Center, Kfar-Saba, Israel

E.D. Ehrenpreis et al. (eds.), *Anal and Rectal Diseases: A Concise Manual*,
DOI 10.1007/978-1-4614-1102-4_8, © Springer Science+Business Media, LLC 2012

Relative Contraindication

Patients with risk factors for incontinence, such as significant diarrhea, preexisting sphincter injuries, or Crohn's disease, should undergo sphincterotomy under very limited circumstances. These patients may benefit from preoperative evaluation with anorectal manometry and/or endoscopic ultrasound. These patients may become incontinent postoperatively or with additional age-related sphincter dysfunction.

Alternatives

Medical treatments for fissure include bulking agents, stool softeners, topical muscle relaxants, or botulinum toxin. Alternative surgical procedures include dilation of the sphincters (largely abandoned) or dermal flap coverage of the fissure. This procedure is generally reserved for patients failing sphincterotomy.

How the Operation Is Performed

Lateral internal sphincterotomy is best performed with the patient in the prone jack-knife position. Preoperative bowel preparation and antibiotics are unnecessary. This procedure may be performed under local, regional, or general anesthesia according to the preference of the patient and surgeon. Anoscopy and proctoscopy are performed for the evaluation of additional anorectal pathology. A 1-cm incision is made overlying the intersphincteric groove (space between the internal and external sphincters) either at the left or the right lateral aspects of the anus. The intersphincteric plane is developed with blunt dissection. A hemostat is used to isolate the internal sphincter, identified by its white appearance. Part of the internal sphincter is divided using sharp dissection or electrocautery. The wound may be left open or closed with sutures. A hypertrophied anal papilla or sentinel pile may be excised at this time. The base of the fissure may be cauterized if there is evidence of recent bleeding.

The length of the internal sphincter incision is dictated by the extent of the fissure. The sphincterotomy should extend into the anal canal up to the same level of the fissure.

Sphincterotomy may also be performed using a "closed" technique. A No 11 blade is inserted into the intersphincteric groove in a parallel manner. Once the tip of the knife has reached the upper level of the incision, the knife is medially rotated to cut the internal sphincter. Care should be taken not to tear the overlying anoderm as it may lead to the development of an anal fistula.

Outcomes

Sphincterotomy is clearly the most definitive treatment available for anal fissure, with permanent healing rates commonly reported to be 95% or greater. The vast majority of fissures will heal within several weeks after surgery.

Complications

Early postoperative complications include anesthetic complications, urinary retention, bleeding, pain, and perianal abscess. The most significant late postoperative complication of sphincterotomy is fecal incontinence. Postoperative incontinence rates have been reported to occur in 0 and 35% of patients. This complication is more common in women than in men. Most patients suffering postoperative incontinence will return to their preoperative status over time. Furthermore, many of these patients will experience minor symptoms only (incontinence to flatus). The rate of major fecal incontinence in selected patients undergoing sphincterotomy by experienced surgeons is actually estimated to be less than 5%.

Warning Signs for Complications

Patients should be monitored for bleeding and abscess formation. Bleeding is typically minor and will resolve spontaneously. Worsening pain, swelling, and purulent drainage are symptoms of abscess and should prompt a return to the surgeon for evaluation. Fecal incontinence in the immediate postoperative period should be treated conservatively with bulking agents, avoidance of dairy products, and a bowel regimen. After complete healing of the surgical wound as well as the fissure, formal evaluation of anorectal function may be required.

Clinical Pearls

Sphincterotomy is a safe operation that affords patients >95% healing of a very painful condition. Patients are rightfully concerned about postoperative incontinence, but can be reassured that the true incidence of permanent, major, postoperative incontinence is low. A trial of medical therapy, along with careful patient selection, will keep this feared complication to a minimum.

Chapter 9
Surgery for Anorectal Abscess

Marc Singer and Shmuel Avital

Description of Procedures

The treatment for perianal abscesses is incision and drainage. This involves opening the skin overlying the abscess to let the pus drain out. Treatment of fistulas or other associated anorectal pathology is deferred until after the infection has been adequately treated.

Indications

The large majority of perianal abscesses should be drained. Small abscesses with minimal symptoms may occasionally be treated with a course of antibiotics.

Contraindications

Patients with large abscesses or a coagulopathy are best treated in the operating room. Patients medically unfit for anesthesia can undergo a bedside or office procedure with local anesthetic.

M. Singer, MD (✉)
Department of Surgery, Division of Colon and Rectal Surgery, NorthShore University
Health System, 2650 Ridge Avenue, Ste 2507, Evanston, IL 60201, USA
e-mail: msinger1@northshore.org

S. Avital, MD
Chief of surgery, Department of Surgery B, Meir Medical Center, Kfar-Saba, Israel

E.D. Ehrenpreis et al. (eds.), *Anal and Rectal Diseases: A Concise Manual*,
DOI 10.1007/978-1-4614-1102-4_9, © Springer Science+Business Media, LLC 2012

Alternatives

Very small abscesses with minimal symptoms may be treated with antibiotics, analgesics, and Sitz™ baths. If resolution or spontaneous drainage occurs, operative drainage may not be necessary. These patients should be monitored very closely for progression of the infectious process, sepsis, or necrotizing infections (Fournier's gangrene).

How the Operation Is Performed

Incision and drainage of perianal abscess is commonly performed in the emergency department, at the bedside, or the outpatient office. A field block is created with local anesthetic such as lidocaine or bupivacaine. If performed in the operating room, then local, regional, or general anesthesia may be used in according to the preference of the patient and surgeon. A scalpel is used to either create a cruciate incision or excise an ellipse of skin overlying the abscess. These techniques will keep the skin open for prolonged drainage. The abscess cavity is copiously irrigated with saline. The cavity should not be packed as this can obstruct the drainage of pus. Dry dressings should be applied and changed frequently to protect the surrounding skin. For very large cavities, a mushroom-tipped catheter can be inserted into the cavity and secured to the skin. This will allow for prolonged drainage as the cavity slowly contracts around the catheter.

Outcomes

Adequate drainage is highly successful in treating the acute infection. Aggressive drainage combined with meticulous wound care will result in healing. However, up to 50% of abscesses may be associated with an anal fistula. At the time of the initial drainage, a fistula may not be apparent. Although fistulotomy at the time of abscess drainage is appropriate in some cases, generally the abscess is treated first, and a fistula is treated subsequently if necessary.

Complications

Early postoperative complications include bleeding, urinary retention, and recurrence of the abscess. Early abscess recurrence may occur when the cavity becomes loculated, all aspects were not thoroughly drained, or the skin closed prematurely. Late recurrence is suggestive of an associated anal fistula and warrants an exam under anesthesia.

Clinical Pearls

A generous incision or excision of skin should be pursued after drainage to assure that the skin remains open for drainage. Packing may obstruct the outflow of pus and should be avoided. Frequent Sitz baths and dressing changes will facilitate the healing processes.

Chapter 10
Surgery for Rectocele

Yehuda Kariv

Definition and Etiology

A rectocele is a herniation of the anterior rectal wall into the posterior wall of the vagina. It is an acquired condition. This herniation begins as a gradual thinning of the rectovaginal septum, first noticeable just above the anal sphincter, and may extend as far as the rectovaginal pouch (Douglas cul-de-sac). A rectocele can be classified as low, midvaginal, or high. Most patients are multiparous. Other predisposing factors include postmenopausal status and hysterectomy. A rectocele can be a cause or a consequence of chronic constipation and is often seen with dyssynergic defecation (paradoxical puborectalis contraction or anismus) and intussusception. Other associated conditions include cystocele (bulging of the bladder into the vagina), enterocele (bulging of the small intestine into the vagina), or uterine prolapse.

Clinical Features and Diagnosis

A small rectocele may cause no signs or symptoms. The larger rectocele may be associated with a multitude of symptoms including difficulty in evacuation, constipation, rectal pain, and rectal bleeding. Patients may have a sensation of a vaginal mass, or protrusion of tissue through the introitus on straining or even while walking. Digitally supporting the perineum or posterior vaginal wall may promote defecation. Straining with defecation may be associated with internal or external rectal prolapse. Associated symptoms also may include fecal incontinence or pruritus.

Y. Kariv, MD (✉)
Tel Aviv Sourasky Medical Center, Colo-rectal Surgery Unit, Division of Surgery,
10 Weizman Street, Tel Aviv, Israel
e-mail: kariv_y@yahoo.com

E.D. Ehrenpreis et al. (eds.), *Anal and Rectal Diseases: A Concise Manual*,
DOI 10.1007/978-1-4614-1102-4_10, © Springer Science+Business Media, LLC 2012

Coexistent anorectal pathology has been noted in up to 80% of patients, with hemorrholds being the most commonly encountered finding.

Diagnosis is usually made by digital vaginal and rectal examinations. Video defecography is useful to rule out other causes of difficult evacuation and to diagnose related conditions (e.g., enterocele, nonrelaxing puborectalis muscle) (see Fig. 2.16). It will show the size of the rectocele as well as the degree to which emptying will occur with defecation. Anal manometry, endorectal ultrasound, and pudendal nerve conduction studies may help in the evaluation of associated sphincter dysfunction. A dynamic MRI is increasingly being used in the work up of pelvic floor dysfunction and may be helpful.

Description of the Procedures

Approaches for rectocele repair include transvaginal, transrectal, transperineal, and abdominal (open or laparoscopic) procedures. Selection of the appropriate procedure depends on associated symptoms, attendant anorectal or gynecological pathologies, and surgeon's preference. Most procedures aim to correct and/or strengthen the rectovaginal septum defect. The most common procedures use the transvaginal or the transanal approach. Other surgical approaches and techniques, such as transperineal repair, site-specific vaginal rectocele repair, or abdominal or laparoscopic rectovaginopexy, are described with comparable results but are less commonly used. Rectocele repair may also be considered in association with perineoplasty in some cases where there is a low presentation secondary to a postobstetric injury with or without an associated low anovaginal fistula. When a high form of a rectocele includes an enterocele, one must consider the transabdominal approach.

Indications

The surgical indications for rectocele repair are controversial. Most surgeons advocate operative repair after failure of conservative measures when a symptomatic rectocele is large, if it fails to empty sufficiently on defecography, or if it is clinically associated with frequent vaginal or perineal manipulation by the patient for satisfactory evacuation, often affecting the patient's quality of life.

Contraindications and Relative Contraindications

Age and/or comorbidity are not an absolute contraindication for surgery. In very high-risk patients, surgery might be contraindicated. When surgery is contraindicated or if the patient refuses an operation, conservative measures should be continued. Transanal approach to rectocele repair may compromise anal sphincter pressures. In patients with anal sphincter dysfunction, alternative approaches should be considered.

Alternatives

Because the usual complaint is difficulty with defecation, the first priority is conservative treatment for the underlying defecation disorder. A fiber-enriched diet, bulk-forming agents, and laxatives should be tried. If a paradoxic contraction of the puborectalis (dyssynergic defecation) is present, biofeedback should be tried before considering surgical repair, though success with this technique is highly variable. A vaginal pessary is a plastic or rubber ring inserted into the vagina to support the bulging tissues. Hormone replacement therapy for postmenopausal women and Kegel exercises may be used to strengthen the pelvic floor muscles.

How the Operation Is Performed

Transvaginal Approach

Rectoceles with accompanying other vaginal defects requiring operative repair, such as cystoceles, enteroceles, or uterine prolapse, are usually best suited for repair through a transvaginal approach. Posterior colporrhaphy is the most commonly performed surgical procedure. The patient is positioned in a dorsal lithotomy position. A longitudinal incision is made in the midline of the posterior vagina wall up to a point above the rectocele, and as far as the fornix when a high rectocele or enterocele is present. Next, the vaginal mucosa is mobilized laterally from the underlying tissues of the rectovaginal septum. Repair includes correction of the septal defect with sutures. Next, the posterior vaginal wall is sutured, once the excess lateral edges of the vaginal mucosa have been trimmed. In addition, correction of the perineum may be performed (perineorrhaphy). Prosthetic meshes to strengthen the rectovaginal septum may reduce the risk of recurrent protrusion and might be used in selected cases.

Transrectal Approach

The transanal approach is ideal for a rectocele associated with dyssynergic defecation. Low- and mid-form rectoceles are best treated with this approach. After placing the patient in a jackknife position and gently introducing the anal retractor, the submucosal plane is infiltrated with a solution of epinephrine 1 per 200,000. After a transverse or a vertical incision, the anterior mucosa and submucosa above the dentate line to the apex of the septal defect are separated from the underlying tissues. The muscular defect in the anterior wall is plicated longitudinally or transversely with absorbable sutures. Excess mucosa is excised and then closed with sutures. Recently, stapled transanal rectal resection (STARR) procedure has gained popularity for rectocele repair when symptoms of obstructive defecation exist. During this procedure, using a specially designed stapler, a transanal circumferential full thickness resection of the distal rectum and anastomosis is performed to remove excessive rectal tissues. Short-term results with this technique are encouraging.

Outcomes

The success rate of surgery is approximately 75%. Vaginal approach might be associated with a lower rate of recurrent rectocele or enterocele than transanal approach. Complications, such as constipation and sexual dysfunction, however, are common and care must be taken when advising surgery. The correlation between symptoms and anatomic defects is weak. Bulging is the principle symptom that correlates with prolapse severity. It is important to determine the prognostic factors. Digital or perineal assistance with defecation might be associated with a favorable outcome, whereas hysterectomy, a large rectocele, use of enemas, and laxatives are associated with a poor result. Slow transit constipation is also associated with a poor outcome. The effect of dyssynergia on surgical outcome is unclear, with better or similar outcome than those without.

Complications

Perioperative mortality is rare and significant morbidity is uncommon. Complications depend on the surgical approach and type of procedure. These may include anesthetic complications, urinary retention, bleeding, pain, infection, anastomotic dehiscence (after STARR procedure), dyspareunia, and mesh erosion.

Warning Signs for Complications

Patients should be monitored for postoperative bleeding and urinary output. Anal or vaginal purulent discharge and fever may signify septic complications.

Clinical Pearls

Definition, etiology, evaluation and management of rectocele are controversial. It is often complicated by other related conditions. Therefore, the management of a patient with a rectocele can be challenging. The importance of a careful and thoughtful preoperative evaluation prior to undertaking operative treatment could not be overemphasized. Unrecognized associated pathologies might jeopardize successful relief of symptoms and therefore should be diagnosed and addressed prior to surgery.

Chapter 11
Surgical Management of Anal Incontinence

Ron Greenberg

Introduction

Fecal incontinence is defined as the involuntary loss of rectal contents (feces, gas) through the anal canal and the inability to postpone an evacuation. Fecal incontinence is very common, estimated prevalence rates are 2–3% with a female/male ratio of 63/37%, with 30% being older than 65 years of age.

Incontinence should be evaluated using an incontinence score to evaluate the severity of the condition and the improvement following any kind of treatment. An acceptable incontinence scoring system is the Wexner incontinence score (see Table 11.1). Fecal incontinence may result from many conditions. These conditions may lead to incontinence related to sphincter innervation injury, direct sphincter muscle damage (internal or external sphincter), weak sphincter muscle and decreased rectal compliance. The most common etiology for fecal incontinence is sphincter damage during vaginal delivery.

Successful management of patients with fecal incontinence depends on a good understanding of the underlying cause that leads to loss of sphincter control. In every patient, a thorough history should be obtained to define the symptoms and their impact. The clinical examination includes a visual inspection, digital rectal examination, and rigid proctoscopy. Colonoscopy should be considered according to routine guidelines. Transanal ultrasound should be performed to assess the presence of a sphincter defect or structural alteration (see Fig. 2.25). Manometry and pudendal nerve terminal motor latency (PTNML) assessment are essential to assess muscle strength, rectal capacity, and pudendal neuropathy. Defecography or dynamic magnetic resonance imaging (MRI) might be also appropriate to evaluate more complex pelvic floor dysfunction.

R. Greenberg, MD (✉)
Surgical Division, Tel Aviv Sourasky Medical Center, 6 Weizman Street, Tel Aviv, Israel
e-mail: rongree@walla.com

E.D. Ehrenpreis et al. (eds.), *Anal and Rectal Diseases: A Concise Manual*,
DOI 10.1007/978-1-4614-1102-4_11, © Springer Science+Business Media, LLC 2012

Table 11.1 Wexner incontinence score

Type of incontinence	Frequency				
	Never	Rarely	Sometimes	Usually	Always
Solid	0	1	2	3	4
Liquid	0	1	2	3	4
Gas	0	1	2	3	4
Wears pad	0	1	2	3	4
Lifestyle alteration	0	1	2	3	4

Never: 0; rarely: <1/month/; sometimes: <1/week, 1/month; usually: <1/day, 1/week; always: 1/ day. 0=perfect continence, 20=complete incontinence

Indications for Surgery

Surgical options should be considered in patients with significant fecal incontinence that is refractory to conservative management. The type of surgical intervention is largely depends on the cause for the incontinence. A full thickness sphincter defect could be primarily repaired while incontinence with an intact sphincter should be approached in another surgical method.

Contraindications

Patients with a low incontinence score should be initially treated with optimal dietary treatment (fiber supplements and antidiarrheal agents) aiming to create bulky stool that is easier to control. Additionally, any causes for diarrhea should be evaluated and treated. Once bowel habits are adequately regulated, some of these patients may not require surgery. Perineal surgery should be cautiously applied to patients with Crohn's disease, as these patients frequently experience prolonged wound healing and aggravation of incontinence.

Alternatives

1. Medical treatment aims at changing the consistency of stool to a firmer stool, resulting in better control over defecation. This should include a high-fiber diet, fiber supplements, and occasionally antidiarrheal drugs.
2. Biofeedback therapy: in this method, patients are trained to improve the strength, the coordination, and the sensation of the rectal ampulla. The patient is connected to a pressure probe in the anus and receives an audio and visual feedback relative to the strength and the proper muscles used for continence. Biofeedback therapy is performed in multiple sessions.
3. A set of exercises for the pelvic and perineal muscles may be employed on a daily basis, improving the strength and coordination of the pelvic muscles and thereby helping in improving incontinence.

How the Operation Is Performed

Various operative approaches are available. Their applicability depends on the individual findings, symptoms, and a clear definition of treatment goals based on the specific findings in the preoperative evaluation.

Sphincter Repair

Anterior Sphincter Repair

Anterior sphincter repair is the most common surgical procedure performed for fecal incontinence. Anterior repair is a good surgical option for incontinent patients with specific damage to the external anal sphincter in its anterior aspect. Most of these patients are women who have suffered obstetric injury following vaginal delivery and development of a scarred area in the anterior part of the anal sphincter muscle. Other causes may be related to trauma or previous anorectal surgery. A good outcome can be expected for most patients following anal sphincter repair; however, long-term function may deteriorate over time. Approximately 80% of patients report satisfactory results 2 years after surgery and 60% after 5 years.

The sphincter defect should not exceed more than 90° based on the endoanal ultrasound findings, as overlapping may become technically impossible. It is important to note that patients with concomitant pudendal neuropathy may also be offered anterior sphincter repair; however, their outcome would be less favorable.

Surgical Technique

The patient is positioned either in a lithotomy position or in a prone jackknife position. A transverse curvilinear incision is then made in the perineum approximately 1 cm from the anodermal junction. A dissection is performed in the recto-vaginal plane, laterally through the ischiorectal fat and up to the levator muscles on both sides. The anoderm is mobilized from the underlying sphincter muscles and scar. Some surgeons may sometimes opt to dissect the intersphincteric groove to repair the internal sphincter separately. Both ends of the external anal sphincter are determined and mobilized enough to perform an overlap. The scar itself is incised in the middle, but is not removed. A levatorplasty is then performed with the aim of helping to lengthen the anal canal by effectively carrying out a posterior colporrhaphy. An overlap repair of the external sphincter is finally performed with good bulk of both ends of the muscle using interrupted sutures.

Postanal Repair

Patients with idiopathic or neurogenic incontinence without an isolated sphincter defect may be suitable candidates for a postanal repair. This procedure consists of a posterior dissection in the intersphincteric groove up to the pelvic floor muscles (levators). The pelvic floor muscles and the external sphincter muscle are then approximated behind the anorectal junction, using either continuous or interrupted sutures. The aim of postanal repair is to restore the anorectal angle, and in this way contribute to improved continence. This procedure is not popular and its success rate is somewhat limited.

Sacral Nerve Stimulation

Sacral nerve stimulation, also known as sacral neuromodulation, involves the implantation of a programmable stimulator subcutaneously, which delivers low-amplitude electrical stimulation via a lead to the sacral nerve, usually accessed via the S3 foramen. In patients with a weak but structurally intact sphincter, it may be possible to alter sphincter and bowel behavior using the surrounding nerves and muscles.

Surgical Technique

Sacral nerve stimulation involves percutaneous application of an electrical current to one of the sacral nerves via an electrode placed through the corresponding sacral foramen. The procedure is generally first tested in patients over a 2–3 week period, with a temporary percutaneous peripheral nerve electrode attached to an external stimulator. If significant benefit is achieved, then the permanent implantable pulse generator is implanted. In patients who have had a permanent implant, complete continence was achieved in more than 40%; in addition, 75–100% of treated patients will experience a decrease of 50% or more in the number of incontinence episodes. There is evidence to suggest an improvement in the ability to defer defecation after permanent implantation. Patients also report improvements in both disease-specific and general quality-of-life scores after this procedure.

The Secca Procedure

The Secca procedure involves controlled radiofrequency (RF) energy delivered to the subcutaneous level of the anal canal (see Fig. 3.13). This submucosal RF energy is delivered circumferentially from below the dentate line and up to the anorectal ring.

The mechanism of action is believed to be related to collagen denaturization, followed by tissue contraction and improved muscle tone. This procedure may be offered to patients with incontinence with no specific anal sphincter defect who have failed conservative treatment. Up to 80% of patients may experience a positive response to this treatment. Clinical studies have shown durable improvement of symptoms over a 5-year period as well as significant improvement in quality-of-life scores.

Surgical Technique

The procedure is performed in the operating room under local anesthesia (see Chap. 24). The patient is placed in the prone jackknife position. A specifically designed anoscope connected to a RF energy source is inserted into the anal canal. A special handle is then pressed, which deploys multiple needles that penetrate the anoderm into the subcutaneous tissue. The needles are deployed circumferentially from a level a few millimeters below the dentate line and up to the anorectal ring.

The RF energy delivery continues for about 45 min with a target temperature of 85°C that is controlled by the Secca system. The needles are then pressed out and the procedure is completed. This procedure is performed on an ambulatory basis. A large multicenter trial demonstrated that the Secca procedure can be safely performed with a negligible complications rate. The Secca procedure significantly improved the Wexner incontinence score and the overall quality of life for most patients having undergone this procedure. Interestingly, with the exception of one center's data, no objective changes were noted in the physiologic studies (manometry, ultrasound, and PNTML) with the exception that resting anal sphincter length increased by 25%.

Injection of Autologous Fat, Silicone, and Collagen

Injection of bulk-enhancing agents into the anal canal area is being evaluated after some successful use in patients with urinary incontinence. This therapy can be performed in an outpatient setting without anesthesia. The bulking agent is usually injected intersphincterically or submucosally. Different agents have been evaluated, including collagen, silicone beads, carbon beads, dextranomer/hyaluronic acid, among others. Results have demonstrated a low complication rate and a mild-to-moderate effect on incontinence symptom improvement.

Implantation of an Artificial Bowel Sphincter

Artificial bowel sphincter was initially developed for the treatment of urinary incontinence. This device has subsequently been modified and adapted for use in the treatment of fecal incontinence.

Surgical Procedure

After perineal dissection, the device is placed around the existing sphincter complex. A tunnel is then constructed to hold a connecting reservoir and pump that controls filling (contraction) and emptying (relaxation) of the sphincter. Reports have demonstrated excellent results with good functional improvement and a significant increase in the patient's quality of life. The success rate has been reported to be approximately 70% of patients retaining a functioning device after implantation. The main complication of this procedure is device infection that leads to device explantation, reported in more than one-third of patients. Patients undergo a trial period of learning to control the sphincter, and most require minor adjustments to the apparatus.

This treatment option is used for end-stage fecal incontinence in selected patients who do not have other treatment options, except for colostomy. The artificial anal sphincter is primarily used at specialist centers or by those surgeons with dedicated interest and experience, because complication rates are substantial, especially in inexperienced hands.

Dynamic Graciloplasty

Muscle transposition of the gracilis muscle was tried initially in the 1950s, but its outcome was limited by the inability to consciously maintain tonic contraction of the neosphincter over long periods of time. This has since been taken over by electrical stimulation of the transposed muscle (dynamic graciloplasty).

Surgical Procedure

Dynamic graciloplasty involves mobilization of the gracilis muscle from the medial leg by detaching it distally at the knee, with a superior-based neurovascular pedicle. This muscle is then tunneled around the existing sphincter complex. An electronic pulse generator applies continuous low-grade current to aid tonic contraction of the muscle. It is thought that this continuous stimulation converts the skeletal muscle fibers of the gracilis to smooth muscle, allowing sustained contraction that aids in continence. Success rates after stimulated graciloplasty have been satisfactory in several studies, but complication rates have been substantial. At present, only a few selected centers perform this procedure, and it is not approved in the United States.

Fecal Diversion

If all other medical and surgical therapies have failed or if comorbidities preclude a more aggressive or time-consuming therapy, the creation of a diverting colostomy remains a valid alternative for patients with severe incontinence (see Chap. 22).

Clinical Pearls

1. Fecal incontinence should be assessed with an incontinence score to obtain a better understanding of the severity of symptoms and, more importantly, as a baseline for further treatment success assessment.
2. Evaluation should consist of anal sphincter ultrasound, nerve conduction studies (PNTML), and anal manometry.
3. Conservative therapy, specifically dietary changes, should be the initial treatment as many patients may improve following this treatment regimen.
4. An area of sphincter muscle defect is a typical finding in women with fecal incontinence following vaginal births. This defect may be approached surgically with anterior sphincter repair with an acceptable success rate.

Chapter 12
Surgery for Hemorrhoids

Marc Singer and Shmuel Avital

Description of the Procedures

There are several surgical procedures available to treat hemorrhoids. The traditional operative management of hemorrhoids is excisional hemorrhoidectomy, that is, surgical removal of hemorrhoid tissue. This operation provides the most definitive control of symptoms, however causes significant postoperative pain. This pain has become notorious and often makes patients reluctant to seek medical attention for hemorrhoids. Several newer techniques were developed in recent years to achieve a less painful postoperative course. These newer alternatives include stapled hemorrhoidopexy, Doppler-guided hemorrhoidal artery ligation (DGHAL), and hemorrhoidectomy using newer energy sources, namely the Ligasure and the Harmonic scalpel.

Stapled hemorrhoidopexy returns prolapsing internal hemorrhoids to the normal anatomic position and secures them in place with surgical staples. Additionally, it interferes with the hemorrhoids' blood supply (Figs. 12.1–12.6). DGHAL involves suturing the internal rectal wall above the dentate line and identifying and ligating all the terminal branches of the superior rectal artery. The ligation results in decongestion of the hemorrhoidal tissue and allows for regeneration of connective tissue within the cushions, thereby facilitating the shrinkage of the internal piles and reduction of the prolapse.

M. Singer, MD (✉)
Department of Surgery, Division of Colon and Rectal Surgery, NorthShore University Health System, 2650 Ridge Avenue, Ste 2507, Evanston, IL 60201, USA
e-mail: msinger1@northshore.org

S. Avital, MD
Chief of surgery, Department of surgery B, Meir Medical Center, Kfar-Saba, Israel

E.D. Ehrenpreis et al. (eds.), *Anal and Rectal Diseases: A Concise Manual*,
DOI 10.1007/978-1-4614-1102-4_12, © Springer Science+Business Media, LLC 2012

In both methods, there are no external incisions, and postoperative pain is dramatically reduced compared to formal excisional hemorrhoidectomy. DGHAL is relatively a new procedure and its long-term success is somewhat inferior to stapled hemorrhoidopexy.

Ligasure hemorrhoidectomy uses a bipolar specifically designed instrument while the Harmonic scalpel uses an ultrasonic device. Both allow simultaneous cutting and sealing of tissues. Postoperative pain is less significant than traditional hemorrhoidectomy.

Indications

The treatment of internal or external hemorrhoids is guided by symptoms. Asymptomatic hemorrhoids are unlikely to create serious risk to patients and should be observed. Definitive treatment of external hemorrhoids can only be accomplished with surgical excision.

Patients with internal hemorrhoids, however, have the option of office-based procedures, such as rubber band ligation, infrared coagulation, or sclerotherapy. Internal hemorrhoids originate proximal to the dentate line, and therefore are not somatically innervated. This allows for the applications of office procedures to internal hemorrhoids with minimal discomfort. Patients who have failed office-based therapies, desire complete treatment at a single setting, or patients on anticoagulation are candidates for excisional hemorrhoidectomy. The indications for stapled hemorrhoidopexy are the same as excisional hemorrhoidectomy, although this operation does not specifically address external hemorrhoids. Patients with symptomatic external hemorrhoids or irreducible internal hemorrhoids are best treated with excision.

Contraindications

Patients with untreated constipation or diarrhea should be optimized medically before surgical therapies are offered. Many of these patients may not require surgery once their bowel habits are adequately regulated, and also a well-managed bowel habit will maximize postoperative outcomes. Hemorrhoidectomy should be cautiously applied to patients with Crohn's disease, as these patients frequently experience prolonged wound healing. Patients with fecal incontinence are at risk of worsening incontinence with any disruption or alteration of sphincter function; therefore, operative therapies should be offered judiciously. Patients with coagulopathy (including those receiving anticoagulants such as warfarin or clopidogrel that cannot be temporarily discontinued) should undergo excisional hemorrhoidectomy, as surgical control of bleeding is the most definitive.

Alternatives

Anal pain after excisional hemorrhoidectomy is intense, prompting many patients to seek alternative therapies. Stapled hemorrhoidopexy is a potential alternative. A newer surgical option is transanal Doppler-guided dearterialization. This surgical technique identifies the arteries supplying the hemorrhoid complexes using a specially designed anoscope/Doppler probe. Sutures are then placed in the anal canal at the locations of the arteries so as to diminish the arterial inflow. At the same time, a suture hemorrhoidopexy is performed. This is a relatively new technique; therefore, long-term clinical outcomes have not been determined.

How the Operation Is Performed

Excisional Hemorrhoidectomy

Excisional hemorrhoidectomy (Ferguson hemorrhoidectomy) is performed in the operating room. Local, regional, or general anesthesia may be used according to patient and surgeon preference. The patient is best positioned in the prone jackknife position to allow maximum exposure of the perineum. The internal and external hemorrhoids are clamped with a hemostat. A suture is placed at the apex of the internal hemorrhoid to devascularize the pedicle and to anchor the closuring suture. A scalpel or cautery is used to create a diamond-shaped incision that encompasses the internal and external hemorrhoidal tissue to be excised. The incision extends widely onto the perineum to allow for smooth closure. Cautery or scissors are used to dissect the hemorrhoidal tissue away from the anus. It is critical to identify the sphincter fibers and carefully sweep them away from the hemorrhoidal tissue to avoid damaging the sphincter. The hemorrhoid is then excised, and the anchoring suture is used to close the resultant defect. This process is repeated a second or third time as needed. The patient can be discharged home postoperatively.

Stapled Hemorrhoidopexy

Patients are prepared and positioned for stapled hemorrhoidopexy as for hemorrhoidectomy. Prolapsing internal hemorrhoids are reduced into the anal canal. A circular anoscope is introduced into the anal canal. A specially designed semicircular anoscope is used to facilitate the placement of a circumferential purse string suture into the mucosa and submucosa proximal to the internal hemorrhoids. A circular stapler is introduced into the anal canal. The purse string is tightened and secured around the stapling device. This draws a circumferential ring of mucosa and submucosa into the head of the stapler. Firing of the stapler simultaneously excises

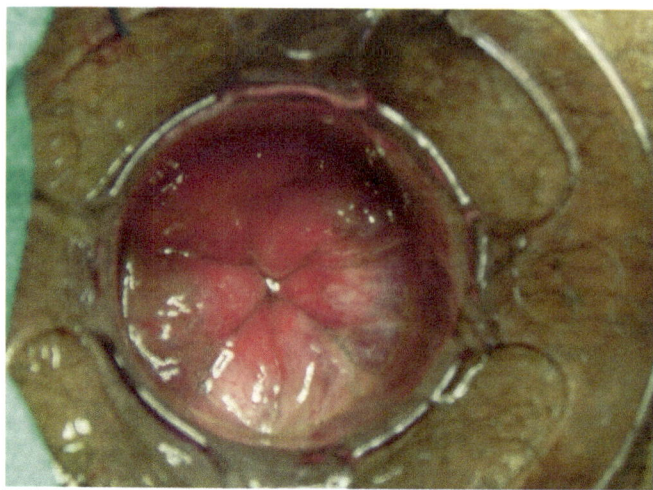

Fig. 12.1 The hemorrhoids can be seen through a special retractor placed in the anal canal

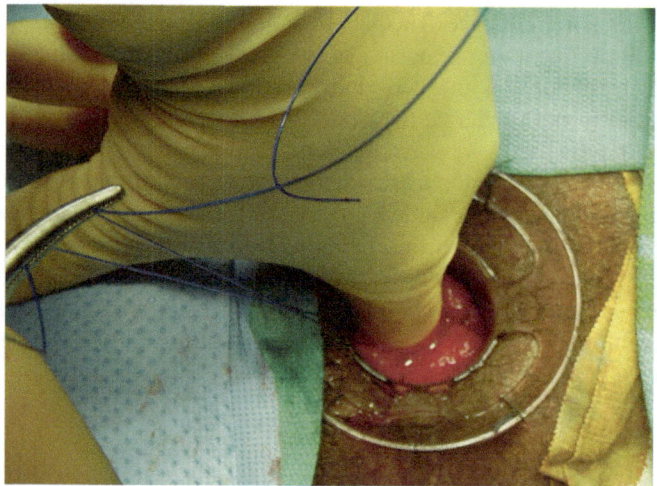

Fig. 12.2 A purse string suture is placed about 2 cm proximal to the dentate line and is tightened around the finger to confirm it is fully circular

this ring of tissue and secures the redundant mucosa/hemorrhoids high in the anal canal with a ring of titanium staples. Although some hemorrhoidal tissue is excised, the operation primary functions as a technique of fixation, reflected by the name "hemorrhoidopexy." There are no external incisions or staples; thus; postoperative pain is reduced (see Figs. 12.1–12.6).

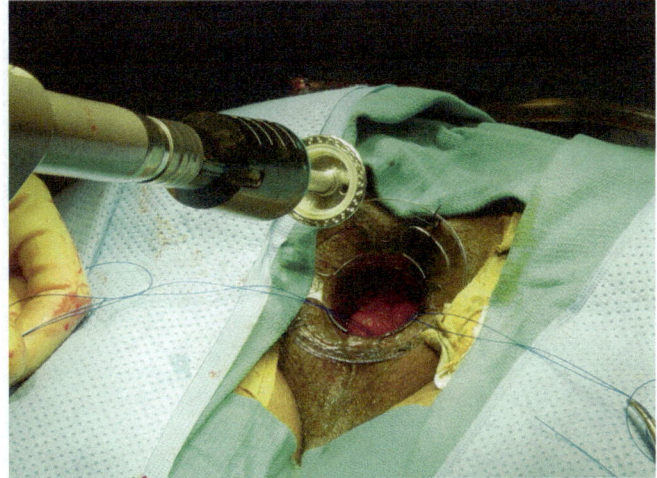

Fig. 12.3 The circular stapler is opened before being inserted into the anorectum

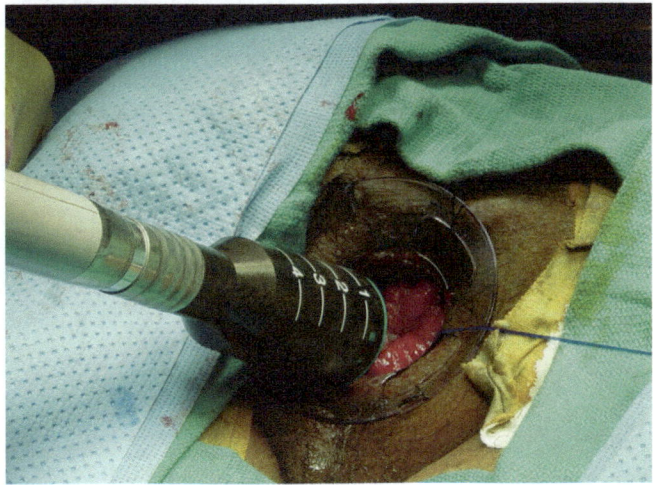

Fig. 12.4 The circular stapler is inserted with the instrument's anvil placed through the purse string

Outcomes

Excisional hemorrhoidectomy remains the gold standard of operative treatment for hemorrhoids. It is more than 95% effective in controlling bleeding, prolapse, and other symptoms, demonstrated on very long-term follow-up. Sustained control of symptoms also depends upon regulation of bowel habits and fiber supplementation.

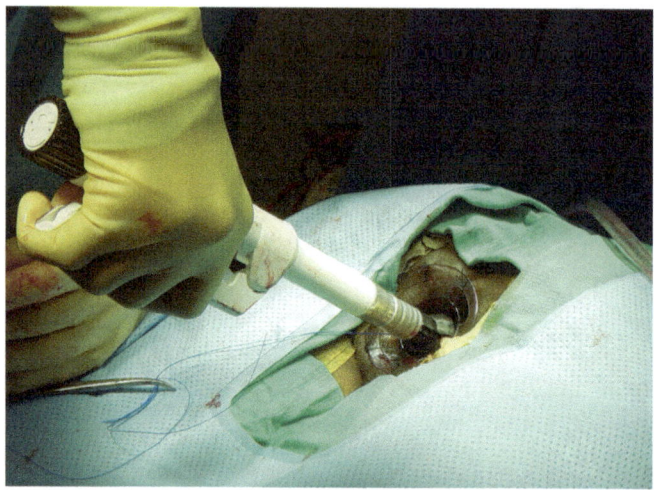

Fig. 12.5 The stapler is closed over the purse string and fired

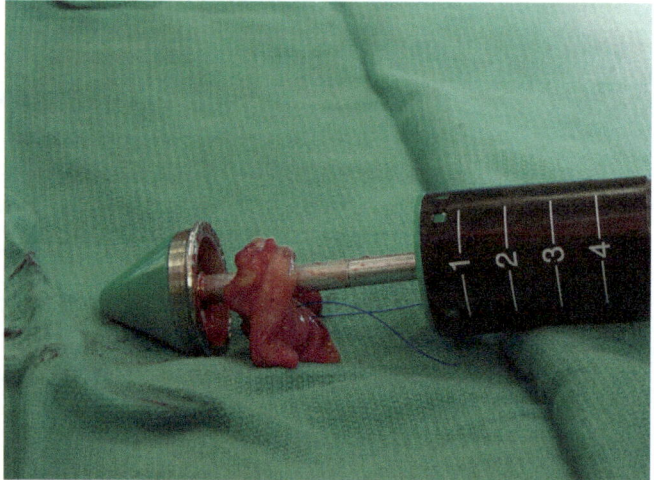

Fig. 12.6 After firing the stapler and its removal, a "doughnut" of tissue including all hemor-rhoidal vessels is retrieved

Stapled hemorrhoidectomy has been demonstrated in multiple clinical trials to be as effective as hemorrhoidectomy, with significantly reduced postoperative pain.

Complications

The primary short-term consideration after hemorrhoidectomy is postoperative pain. Even in the absence of complications, the suture lines in exquisitely sensitive ano-derm cause severe pain. Other postoperative complications include bleeding, urinary retention, fecal impaction, and abscess. Late postoperative complications include nonhealing wounds, fistulas, anal stenosis, and fecal incontinence. The complications of stapled hemorrhoidopexy are similar, but also carry some very rare complications related to the staple line, such as development of a rectovaginal fistula.

Warning Signs for Complications

A small amount of postoperative bleeding is normal. Massive bleeding should prompt immediate return to the hospital. The triad of fever, pain, and urinary retention can signify evolving pelvic sepsis and warrants a return visit to the surgeon.

Clinical Pearls

Hemorrhoids are an extremely common clinical problem. Fortunately, very few patients with hemorrhoids require surgical treatment. As hemorrhoids are a benign process, treatment should be symptom directed. An attempt at dietary changes and fiber supplementation is suggested as an initial step for all patients. Medical therapy is also recommended (see Chap. 3, Section "Hemorrhoids"). Depending on symptom severity, office-based treatments can often be attempted, prior to performing surgical treatments for refractory patients. Patients should be informed that hemorrhoidectomy is a safe and highly effective operation, but that postoperative pain is significant. Newer surgical alternatives should be considered if available.

Chapter 13
Surgery for Hidradenitis Suppurativa

Marc Singer and Shmuel Avital

Description of Procedures

If a subcutaneous abscess is present, then incision and drainage can be performed to drain the acute infections. Definitive management can only be accomplished with full-thickness excision of the affected skin. Drainage, debridements, and other local procedures are appropriate to manage symptoms or acute infections; however, the only curative option is complete excision of the skin.

Indications

Acute infection in the setting of hidradenitis will manifest as subcutaneous abscesses. A very small abscess that does not cause significant pain may be managed with antibiotics and local measures (warm compresses). However, most abscesses will cause pain, drainage, and a foul odor, and therefore should be treated with surgical drainage. When a region of hidradenitis can no longer be managed with drainage and debridement, or the patient desires definitive management, then full-thickness excision of the affected skin should be performed. In addition, very long standing disease (20–30 years) presents a low, but not insignificant, risk of squamous cell carcinoma. This risk factor warrants the complete excision of a tissue bed with chronic disease.

M. Singer, MD (✉)
Department of Surgery, Division of Colon and Rectal Surgery, NorthShore University Health System, 2650 Ridge Avenue, Ste 2507, Evanston, IL 60201, USA
e-mail: msinger1@northshore.org

S. Avital, MD
Chief of Surgery, Department of Surgery B, Meir Medical Center, Kfar-Saba, Israel

E.D. Ehrenpreis et al. (eds.), *Anal and Rectal Diseases: A Concise Manual*,
DOI 10.1007/978-1-4614-1102-4_13, © Springer Science+Business Media, LLC 2012

Contraindications

Drainage of subcutaneous abscesses is a relatively minor procedure and therefore appropriate for nearly all patients. If regional or general anesthesia were required, then only contraindications to anesthesia would prevent the procedure. Anticoagulation (Coumadin, Plavix) would make drainage in the operating room safer as definitive control of bleeding can be accomplished.

Full-thickness excision of affected skin is contraindicated in patients medically unfit for anesthesia. In addition, access to appropriate postoperative wound care should be considered. Wound care and dressing changes of the perianal and perineal regions commonly require assistance, and a lack thereof should be considered a relative contraindication.

Alternatives

Treatment with systemic antibiotics may be helpful for small and minimally symptomatic abscesses. In addition, chronic antibiotic therapy can be used to suppress infections, thus delaying the time interval between surgical procedures. Tetracycline has been the most widely evaluated drug for this purpose, but many broad-spectrum antibiotics have been successfully used in this fashion. Patients should be reminded that antibiotics are one component of symptom management and do not represent a cure.

How the Operation Is Performed

Simple incisions may be performed in the office setting with local anesthesia. The skin is cleansed with an iodine solution or chlorhexidine. Lidocaine or bupivacaine is infiltrated to create a field block surrounding the abscess. A scalpel is used to open the cavity and associated subcutaneous fistulas. The wound is generously irrigated with saline to remove pus or devitalized tissue. Wounds are left open to drain.

More extensive regions of hidradenitis may require drainage procedures in the operating room. Local, regional, or general anesthesia may be employed according to the judgment of the patient and surgeon. In the operating room, the patients can be sedated and more aggressively anesthetized compared to an office setting. This allows the surgeon to unroof all abscess cavities and debride the cavities and fistulous tracks with curettage. The surgeon should carefully and meticulously explore all cavities with a probe to identify and open and subcutaneous fistulas.

For a curative approach, full-thickness excision of the affected skin is performed in the operating room. This can be also performed under local, regional, or general anesthesia depending on the extent of disease and the patient and surgeon preference. Full-thickness skin, including associated skin structures, such as hair follicles and apocrine sweat glands, must be excised down to normal subcutaneous fat. As hidradenitis is a skin disease, it is unnecessary to excise the underlying muscular fascia, periosteum, or anal mucosa. Deep margins should be soft, normal subcutaneous fat. Lateral margins should be reasonably soft skin, understanding that recurrence at those lateral margins is always a risk. If extensive perianal disease is present, then a staged operation may be required. Circumferential excision of the perianal skin can lead to anal stenosis.

Wounds may be closed primarily if possible, or left open to granulate. Aggressive wound care, including frequent Sitz baths, whirlpool therapy, or in some circumstances negative pressure wound management systems can achieve excellent results. If the wounds are clean, with minimal infection or inflammation at the time of excision, then immediate skin grafting may be performed. Skin grafting may accelerate the time to healing. However, perianal skin grafts have a high failure rate and may lead to stricturing. Therefore, grafting should be reserved for perineal and buttock disease.

Outcomes

Since hidradenitis is limited to the skin, excision does not typically result in any long-term dysfunction. Recurrence of infection is the primary outcome measure of clinical significance. Recurrence occurs either within the site of excision or remotely. Recurrence at the deep margin is due to partial thickness excision, which is inadequate. The hidradenitis may reoccur at the margin of excision. This is not necessarily a failure of treatment. It may represent a progression of disease. In fact, judicious excision is advisable in many circumstances, rather than extending the excision to include visibly normal skin, which results in larger open wounds or skin grafts. Of course, recurrence at distant sites (axilla, scalp) is possible, and is unrelated to treatment of perianal or perineal disease.

Complications

Early complications of full-thickness skin excision include bleeding, pain, or infection. Infection is relatively rare if the wounds are left open. The usual complications of perianal operations also include urinary retention, fecal impaction, sphincter spasm, etc. If skin grafts are employed, then graft failure, recurrence under the graft, or donor site complications (pain, bleeding) are possible.

Warning Signs for Complications

Early postoperative bleeding will be readily apparent to patients. Fevers, urinary retention, worsening pain, purulent drainage, or failure to evacuate stool within 3–5 days may indicate infection.

Clinical Pearls

Management with local measures such as unroofing and curettage are reasonable management options. It is imperative that patients understand that these are part of a management process and not curative. Patients should be informed early in their clinical course that full-thickness excision might ultimately become necessary. Depending on the extent of disease, this may involve a massive open perineal wound. Patients should make psychological preparations, employ home health care, or even an inpatient stay in a wound care facility as necessary. Meticulous wound care should include frequent baths or showers, ideally in a whirlpool tub. In addition, strict management of the bowel habit with bulking agents to facilitate perineal hygiene is necessary. Diarrhea will not allow for appropriate cleansing.

Chapter 14
Surgery for Anorectal Fistula

Marc Singer and Shmuel Avital

Introduction

Anorectal fistulas most often result from an infectious process of an anal gland situated at the dentate line. Other causes of anorectal fistulas are Crohn's disease, trauma, anal fissure, cancer, radiation, and specific infections (actinomycosis, tuberculosis, and Chlamydia). Fistulas are classified based on the course of their tract. A simple classification divides anorectal fistulas into simple or complex. Fistulas with subcutaneous, intersphincteric, or low transsphincteric tracts are considered simple. Complex fistulas are those with high transsphincteric, supra or extra sphincteric tracts, and have multiple tracts or are recurrent.

There are multiple surgical procedures for anorectal fistulas. The choice of a procedure is based on the nature of the fistula and the surgeon preference. The success of a procedure is evaluated by the recurrence rate and the impact on continence.

Description of Procedures

Fistulotomy remains the "gold standard." This operation involves opening of the fistula track and allowing it to granulate closed over time. Other choices, which do not involve division of sphincter muscle, include mucosal advancement flaps,

M. Singer, MD (✉)
Department of Surgery, Division of Colon and Rectal Surgery, NorthShore University Health System, 2650 Ridge Avenue, Ste 2507, Evanston, IL 60201, USA
e-mail: msinger1@northshore.org

S. Avital, MD
Chief of Surgery, Department of Surgery B, Meir Medical Center, Kfar-Saba, Israel

E.D. Ehrenpreis et al. (eds.), *Anal and Rectal Diseases: A Concise Manual*,
DOI 10.1007/978-1-4614-1102-4_14, © Springer Science+Business Media, LLC 2012

dermal advancement flaps, fibrin sealant injection, collagen plug insertion, and placement of permanent or cutting setons. Recently, a new and promising technique was introduced—ligation of intersphincteric fistula tract (LIFT).

Indications

In medically fit patients, all fistulas should be treated, as they eventually lead to chronic drainage, perianal skin irritation, and recurrent abscess formation. Fistulotomy is best employed for intersphincteric or low transsphincteric fistulas, as only a small amount of the external sphincter will need to be divided. High transsphincteric, suprasphincteric, and extrasphincteric fistulas should be considered for alternative procedures that do not involve division sphincter fibers.

Contraindications

Fistulotomy involves division of sphincter muscle. Patients with impaired continence, or those at high risk of incontinence (chronic diarrhea, previous fistulotomy, obstetric sphincter injury, Crohn's disease), should undergo fistulotomy under very limited circumstances. Only a minimal amount of muscle should be divided in these patients, and alternative surgical techniques should be considered. Additionally, anterior fistulas in women represent a high-risk fistula due to the relative paucity of sphincter muscle mass at this location.

Alternatives

There are several surgical alternatives to fistulotomy. These include mucosal advancement flaps, dermal advancement flaps, fibrin sealant injection, collagen plug injection, permanent or cutting seton placement, and the LIFT procedure.

How the Operation Is Performed

Fistulotomy may be performed with local, regional (spinal), or general anesthesia according to the preferences of the patient and surgeon. Preoperative bowel preparation or antibiotics are not necessary. The patient is best positioned in the prone jackknife position with the buttocks taped widely apart to allow maximum exposure of the perineum. Formal anoscopy and proctoscopy are performed to evaluate the anus and rectum for additional pathology or inflammatory changes. The external fistula

Fig. 14.1 The external fistula opening is cannulated with a specialized fistula probe to demonstrate a communication into the anal canal. If the internal opening cannot be identified, then the external opening may be flushed with saline or hydrogen peroxide to aid the identification of the internal opening. Additional tracks or side branches must be identified as well. The fistulotomy is performed by dividing the skin, fat, and muscle tissue overlying the probe. This can be accomplished with scalpel or electrocautery

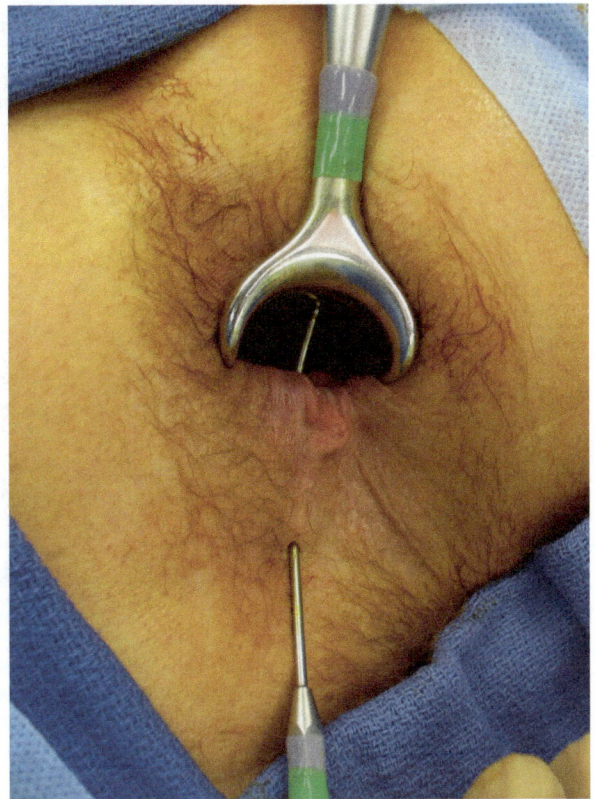

opening is cannulated with a specialized fistula probe to demonstrate a communication into the anal canal. If the internal opening cannot be identified, then the external opening may be flushed with saline or hydrogen peroxide to aid the identification of the internal opening. Additional tracks or side branches must be identified as well. The fistulotomy is performed by dividing the skin, fat, and muscle tissue overlying the probe. This can be accomplished with scalpel or electrocautery. Patients may be discharged home postoperatively (Fig. 14.1).

If the fistula track encircles too much sphincter muscle to safely perform a fistulotomy (concern for postoperative incontinence), then an indwelling seton should be placed at that time. The seton may be made from a Silastic vessel loop or a permanent suture (silk). It is tied loosely to itself. This will function as a drain, maintaining patency of the external opening so as to drain infection and to prevent abscess formation. This may be used as a bridge until the patient and surgeon are prepared for alternative procedures. In the highest risk patients, the seton may be a permanent option (Fig. 14.2).

The LIFT procedure is performed by dissection in the intersphincteric plain toward the fistulous tract, following probing of the fistula. Once the surgeon has

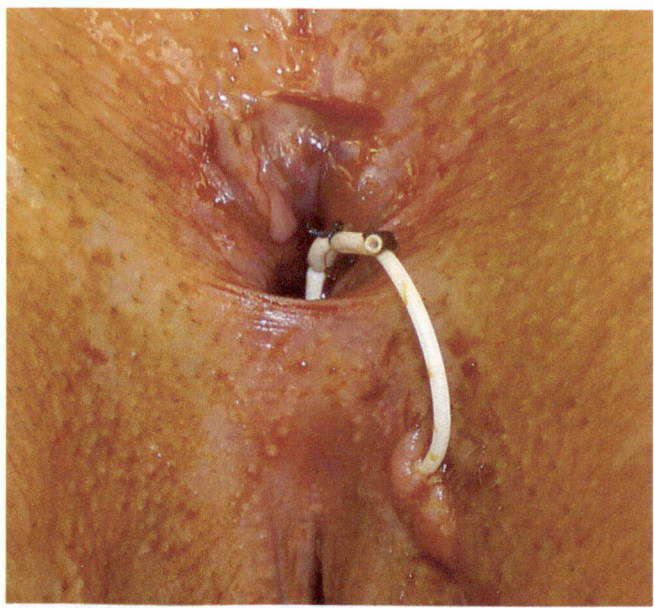

Fig. 14.2 If the fistula track encircles too much sphincter muscle to safely perform a fistulotomy (concern for postoperative incontinence), then an indwelling seton should be placed at that time. The seton may be made from a Silastic vessel loop or a permanent suture (silk). It is tied loosely to itself. This will function as a drain, maintaining patency of the external opening so as to drain infection and to prevent abscess formation. This may be used as a bridge until the patient and surgeon are prepared for alternative procedures. In the highest risk patients, the seton may be a permanent option

reached the tract, it is ligated on both sides (the internal anal sphincter and the external anal sphincter) and transected. The intersphincteric tract is removed, and the external tract is cleansed and left open for drainage.

Outcomes

Fistulotomy is successful in permanently treating fistulas for more than 95% of cases. It is highly effective and safe. Fistulotomy represents the most definitive and successful treatment for anal fistula.

Mucosal and dermal flaps have been reported to have an approximate 80% success rate. Fibrin sealant and collagen plugs have widely variable healing rates, but are typically between 40 and 50% successful. A loose or draining seton is not a curative procedure. Instead, it is a permanent management option or an intermediate step in preparation for additional procedures. Initial results for the LIFT procedure are promising, although larger series are needed to evaluate the success rate.

Complications

Early complications include bleeding, pain, and urinary retention. Late complications include sphincter dysfunction resulting in fecal incontinence. Reported rates of incontinence range from 0 to 45%. As the surgical technique is rather straightforward, this huge variability likely reflects differences in patient selection. Most incontinence is temporary and minor. If significant fecal incontinence persists, then sphincteroplasty is a potential option to restore function.

Warning Signs for Complications

Patients who cannot urinate for 6 h after surgery may be experiencing urinary retention and should be evaluated immediately. Ongoing bleeding beyond spotting on the dressings should prompt a return visit. Postoperative pain is normal, but worsening pain may signify that an abscess has developed. Postoperative incontinence should be reported to the surgeon, and often the symptoms can be managed medically.

Clinical Pearls

Although there has been a decrease in the number of fistulotomies performed at many centers, this surgery continues to be the most commonly performed operation for anorectal fistula. Patients with intersphincteric and low transsphincteric fistulas are the best candidates for fistulotomy. High transsphincteric, suprasphincteric, and extrasphincteric fistulas represent a high risk for postoperative incontinence. Patients with HIV, Crohn's disease, chronic diarrhea, and anterior fistulas in women should also be considered high risk. If fistulotomy is not suitable, then drainage with a seton for 6–12 weeks prior to additional treatment will minimize infection/inflammation and maximize successful outcomes. It is important for patients and surgeons to accept at the onset that safe treatment for anal fistula may be an ongoing process, including multiple trips to the operating room. This is best viewed as an investment in a good long-term outcome that balances closure of the fistula and preservation of continence.

Chapter 15
Surgery for Rectal Prolapse

Yehuda Kariv

Definition and Clinical Features

Complete or full-thickness rectal prolapse is defined as protrusion of the entire rectal wall through the anal canal. Symptoms may include bowel protrusion during lifting or coughing, need for manual replacement, mucous discharge, and rectal bleeding. Fecal incontinence and/or constipation are frequently associated with rectal prolapse. Fecal incontinence may be related to stretch injury to the anal sphincter muscles, and/or pudendal and perineal nerves. Incarcerated rectal prolapse is an uncommon complication and may lead to bowel strangulation.

Description of the Procedures

The goals of surgery are to prevent recurrent prolapse and improve continence and bowel function with acceptable morbidity and recurrence rates. Numerous procedures have been described for the treatment of rectal prolapse and are generally categorized as *abdominal* or *perineal* approaches. *Abdominal access* is possible through either an open incision or laparoscopy. Abdominal procedures usually involve fixation of the rectum. Colonic resection during an abdominal procedure is frequently considered in patients with redundant sigmoid colon or significant constipation to prevent exacerbation or new onset constipation. *Perineal procedures* involve resection or plication of redundant bowel.

Y. Kariv, MD (✉)
Tel Aviv Sourasky Medical Center, Colo-rectal Surgery Unit, Division of Surgery,
10 Weizman Street, Tel Aviv, Israel
e-mail: kariv_y@yahoo.com

E.D. Ehrenpreis et al. (eds.), *Anal and Rectal Diseases: A Concise Manual*,
DOI 10.1007/978-1-4614-1102-4_15, © Springer Science+Business Media, LLC 2012

Indications

Symptoms and complications of rectal prolapse frequently worsen with time. Therefore, complete or full-thickness rectal prolapse is an indication for surgery unless contraindications exist. The general health of the patient is of great importance in the preoperative decision making. Abdominal procedures are ideal for young, fit patients, whereas perineal procedures are reserved for older, frail patients with significant comorbidities. Acute incarcerated rectal prolapse may frequently be reduced; however, emergency resection is occasionally indicated.

Contraindications and Relative Contraindications

Age and/or comorbidity are not an absolute contraindication for surgery. In frail elderly patients, a perineal approach is usually safe. In very high-risk patients, any surgical procedure may be contraindicated.

Alternatives

When surgery is contraindicated or if the patient refuses an operation, noninvasive approaches and limited office-based procedures may be employed. These include correction of constipation, perineal strengthening exercises, manual anal support during defecation, and adhesive strapping of buttocks and other. Rubber band ligation, injection of a sclerosing agent, or infrared coagulation of redundant rectal tissue may offer some degree of palliation in cases of incomplete rectal prolapse.

How the Operation Is Performed

Abdominal repairs usually involve mobilization of the rectum and its fixation to the sacrum with sutures or a prosthetic material or mesh. Many abdominal techniques have been described, differing in the extent of rectal mobilization, the methods used for rectal fixation, and the inclusion or exclusion of bowel resection. The abdomen can be approached through an open incision or laparoscopy. Open incisions usually include a midline laparotomy or a transverse suprapubic (Pfannenstiel) incision. The rectum is usually mobilized by dissecting posteriorly in the presacral space down to the pelvic floor; however, the extent of lateral dissection is controversial. Suture rectopexy usually involves securing the posterior rectal wall or intact lateral ligaments to the periosteum of the sacrum with nonabsorbable sutures. In anterior mesh repair, such as the *Ripstein procedure*, the mesh is wrapped around the anterior aspect of the rectum and fixed on both sides of the sacral promontory. In posterior mesh repairs, such as the *Wells procedure*, the mesh is placed behind the rectum and superior rectal artery and fixed to the sacrum, before being wrapped around both sides and fixed to the lateral mesorectum. Anterior wraps may be complicated with stenosis and fixation, and therefore, most authors prefer posterior repairs when mesh is selected for rectal fixation.

Compared with laparotomy, laparoscopic rectopexy has the potential advantages of reduced pain, shortened hospital stay, early recovery, and early return to work. The procedure involves either suture or posterior mesh rectopexy, with or without resection. Sigmoid colon resection is well suited for patients with rectal prolapse, a long redundant sigmoid, and a long history of constipation. The addition of sigmoid resection to rectopexy (resection rectopexy; *Frykman–Goldberg procedure*) may improve postoperative constipation.

Perineal procedures may be performed in either lithotomy or a prone jackknife position. The *Delorme operation* involves submucosal dissection to separate the mucosa from the sphincter and the muscularis propria starting with a circumferential incision made 1 cm proximal to the dentate line. The mucosa is stripped to the apex of the protruding bowel. The redundant mucosa is excised and the denuded muscularis propria is plicated like an accordion. The edges of the mucosa are then sutured. This procedure has an additional advantage of excision of a concomitant rectal ulcer if present. The Delorme procedure represents a surgical alternative for patients with prolapse who may be unable to tolerate a more extensive operation, such as the elderly, frail patients, and those who are medically unfit for major surgery. During perineal rectosigmoidectomy (*Altmeier operation*), the prolapsed rectum is exteriorized. A circumferential incision is made through all layers of the bowel 1 cm proximal to the dentate line. The prolapsed bowel is delivered. The peritoneal cavity is entered by incising the peritoneum anteriorly at the pouch of Douglas. Any redundant colon is delivered through the defect and resected. The peritoneum is closed and a coloanal anastomosis is completed. Anterior or posterior levator ani muscle plication (levatorplasty) might be added to reduce recurrence rates and improve continence. An *Altmeier* procedure might have better results than *Delorme operation* with lower recurrence rates and better functional outcomes. Therefore, it is often suggested as the best operation for elderly patients or individuals with profound comorbidity, in whom an abdominal procedure might be contraindicated. It is also suitable for elderly or high-risk patients with incontinence because a concomitant levatorplasty can be performed. This operation remains the ideal option for patients presenting with an incarcerated, gangrenous prolapse. The *Thiersch procedure*, which entails encircling the anal canal using a wire, tape, or mesh, does not eradicate prolapse but merely prevents its further descent by providing mechanical support, and hence, it is associated with a high recurrence rate. Given the safety of modern anesthetic techniques, it is rarely used in patients with rectal prolapse.

Outcomes

Variable recurrence rates have been reported after both abdominal and perineal repairs. Five to ten percent recurrence rates after abdominal procedures and 10–20% after perineal procedures are considered acceptable.

Improvement in bowel function including fecal incontinence and constipation is highly variable and may depend on the method of repair and associated procedures. Improvement of continence in at least 50% of patients is usually reported after most types of operations. The addition of a sigmoid colon resection may improve constipation in selected cases.

Complications

Mortality rates after surgery for rectal prolapse range from 0 to 3% in most series. In elderly and/or high-risk patients, mortality is uncommon if patients and procedures are carefully selected. Complications depend on the type of surgical procedure. These may include anesthetic complications, urinary retention, bleeding, pain, anastomotic dehiscence when bowel is resected and anastomosed, presacral hematoma after rectopexy, and stenosis and constipation after anterior mesh procedures. Bowel function and continence should be observed for improvement for 6–12 months after surgery. Residual complaints should then be treated conservatively or surgically.

Warning Signs for Complications

Patients should be monitored for postoperative bleeding. Ileus, fever, anal purulent discharge, and abdominal tenderness may signify septic complications.

Clinical Pearls

Multiple surgical procedures for rectal prolapse exist, and there is no clear predominant treatment of choice. Abdominal procedures are ideal for young, fit patients, whereas perineal procedures are reserved for older, frail patients with significant comorbidities. The choice of operation depends also on the surgeon's preference and experience. Results after all abdominal procedures are comparable. Laparoscopic rectopexy has results equivalent to those of open rectopexy. Laparoscopy may enhance postoperative recovery compared with an open approach. Perineal procedures are useful for patients who are not fit for abdominal procedures. Careful selection of patients and surgical procedures are crucial for optimization of outcomes.

Chapter 16
Surgery for Rectovaginal Fistula

Marc Singer and Shmuel Avital

Description of Procedures

There are several treatment options available for the treatment of rectovaginal fistula (RVF). The appropriate choice depends upon the etiology of the fistula, the specific location of the fistula, if there is sphincter injury, and the patient's symptoms.

The types of repair may be divided into local or abdominal. Local repairs include excision with layers, endorectal advancement flap with or without sphincteroplasty, labial fat pad flap (Martius flap or bulbocavernosus flap, see Figs. 16.1–16.7), among others. Abdominal repairs include division of the fistula and interposition of healthy tissue or proctectomy with coloanal anastomosis. These two approaches may require the use of healthy tissue for transposition.

Recent reports have described the use of biomaterials for closure of RVFs, mainly collagen plugs. The main advantage of this technique is that no surgical incision is required, since the plug is inserted and secured to the fistulous tract. This is a significant advantage for patients with Crohn's disease. Success may be achieved with this technique in more than 50% of patients, and the risk for complications is negligible.

Generally, the most common operation performed by colon and rectal surgeons is the endorectal advancement flap. This technique involves the mobilization of healthy rectal tissue to cover the fistula.

M. Singer, MD (✉)
Department of Surgery, Division of Colon and Rectal Surgery, NorthShore University Health System, 2650 Ridge Avenue, Ste 2507, Evanston, IL 60201, USA
e-mail: msinger1@northshore.org

S. Avital, MD
Chief of Surgery, Department of Surgery B, Meir Medical Center, Kfar-Saba, Israel

E.D. Ehrenpreis et al. (eds.), *Anal and Rectal Diseases: A Concise Manual*,
DOI 10.1007/978-1-4614-1102-4_16, © Springer Science+Business Media, LLC 2012

Indications

All symptomatic fistulas should be treated. The typical symptoms are drainage of stool, mucus, or air per vagina. In addition, women may experience vaginitis, urinary tract infections, dyspareunia, etc. Occasionally, a woman may have a tiny RVF that remains asymptomatic. This does not necessarily require treatment; however, this is an unusual scenario.

A fistula due to an obstetric injury can generally be treated with an endorectal advancement flap alone. However, a fistula in the setting of fecal incontinence is best treated with endorectal advancement flap combined with a sphincteroplasty. Radiation-induced fistulas are difficult to treat due to radiation injury of the surrounding tissues. An attempt at local repair is may be tried, but high rates of recurrence may necessitate the performance of a proctectomy and a coloanal anastomosis. Recurrent fistulas may require fecal diversion or interposition flaps to provide healthy, well-vascularized tissue between the rectum and vagina.

Contraindications

Patients medically unfit for anesthesia may be managed with bulking agents and strict attention to perineal hygiene. Inflammatory bowel disease or diarrhea should be adequately controlled prior to surgical therapy.

Alternatives

Patients unfit for operations or electing not to undergo surgical repair may be managed symptomatically. Bulking agents will minimize liquid stool draining through the fistula. Strict attention is given to perineal hygiene. Vaginal irrigation may be required. Fecal diversion (ileostomy or colostomy) will prevent drainage of stool through an RVF, but will not necessarily prevent drainage of mucus or vaginal irritation.

How the Operation Is Performed

The endorectal advancement flap is performed with local, regional, or general anesthesia depending on the preference of the patient and surgeon. The patient is best positioned in the prone jackknife position to allow for maximal visualization of the anterior anorectal wall. The fistula is carefully probed to define the anatomy and

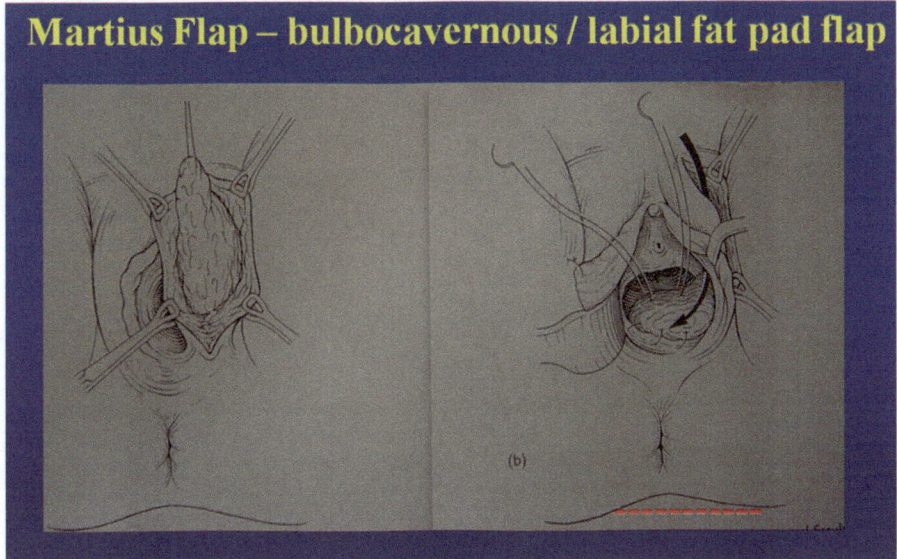

Fig. 16.1   A schematic drawing of the labial fat pad flap

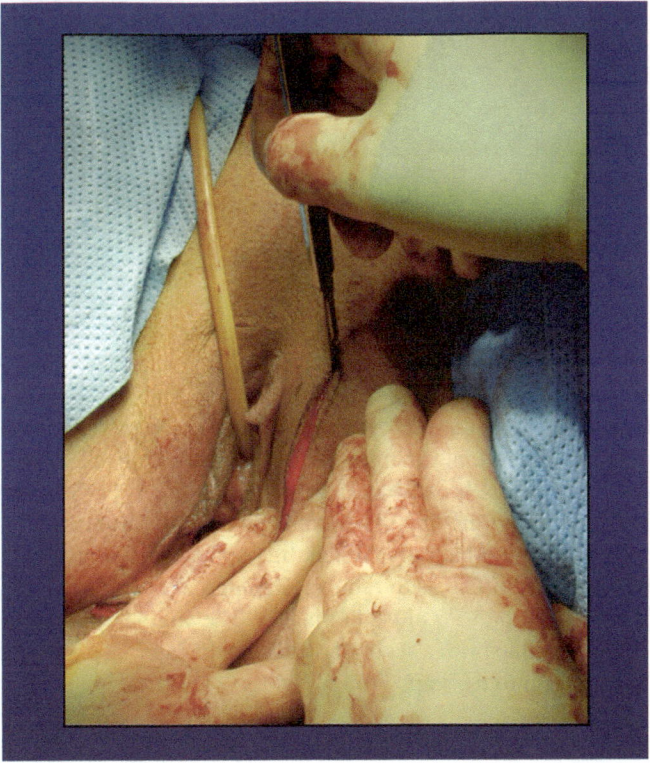

Fig. 16.2   Patient in a lithotomy position. A longitudinal skin incision over the labia majora

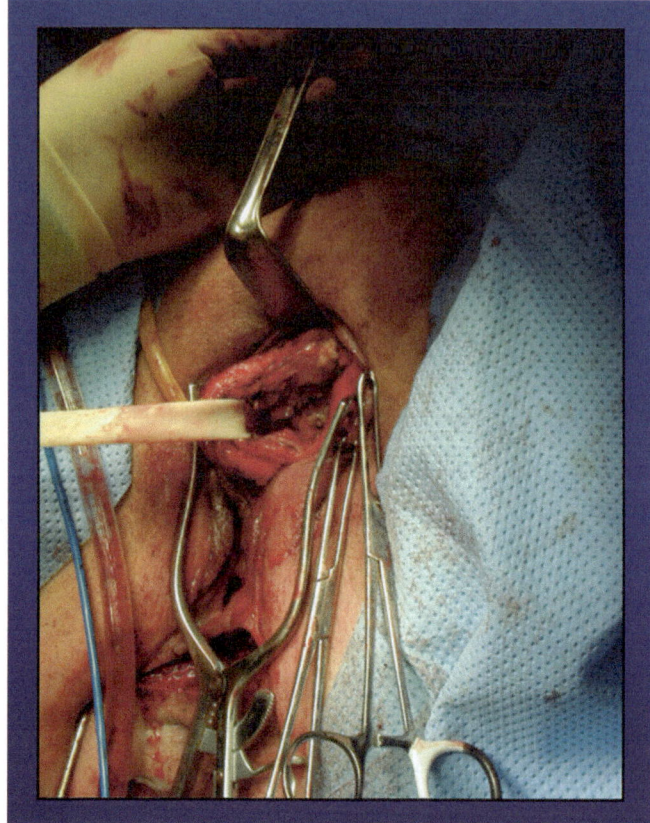

Fig. 16.3 Dissection of the perineum between the anal canal and the vagina and dissection of the labial fat pad

confirm there are no side branches of the fistula or undrained abscess cavities. Local anesthetic is injected into the rectovaginal septum prior to separation of the RV septum with hydrodissection. An incision is then made distal to the fistula and extended laterally. A wide, broad-based flap is necessary to ensure adequate blood supply to the distal end of the flap. The flap is generously mobilized in the submucosal plane proximally and laterally. When the flap has been completely mobilized, the distal tip is debrided off so as to remove the internal opening. The fistula is then cored out and the RV septum is closed in layers. The vaginal aspect of the fistula is left open to drain. The flap is then secured overlying the internal opening. Absorbable sutures are used to secure the flap.

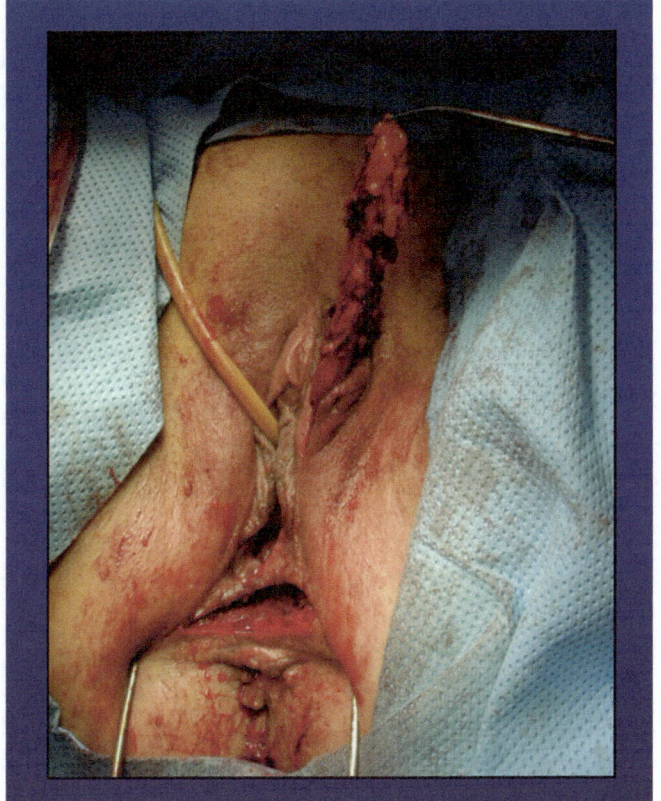

Fig. 16.4 Cutting the lower end of the labial fat pad

If a sphincter defect is present on physical exam and/or endoscopic ultrasound, a concomitant overlapping sphincteroplasty should be performed at this same operative setting. The flap can then be advanced over the repair and closed.

Outcomes

The success rate of mucosal flaps to treat RVF is approximately 75%. Surgical failure will result in a persistent or recurrent fistula. If one technique fails, then an alternative technique should be considered for subsequent repairs. In addition, consideration for a proximal diverting stoma should be included in the discussion of surgical planning with the patient. If a stoma is constructed, the secondary repair

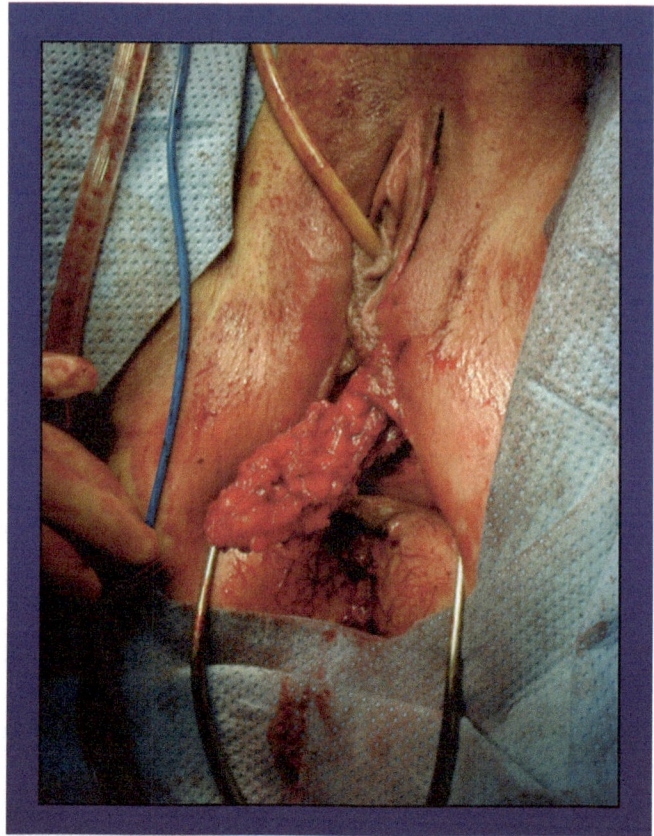

Fig. 16.5 Passing the fat pad through a tunnel into the rectovaginal plane

should be performed, and the stoma closed approximately 3 months after the repair has been deemed successful.

Complications

The most common complication of RVF repair is breakdown of the flap. Failure of the flap may be due to ischemia, tension on the flap or bleeding deep to the flap. If the flap is too thin, the vascular supply in the mucosa only will be inadequate to fully heal the repair. If the flap is under tension, then healing will also be compromised. Abscess, urinary retention, and pain are possible as with all anorectal operations. Late complications include dyspareunia, late recurrence, and fecal incontinence.

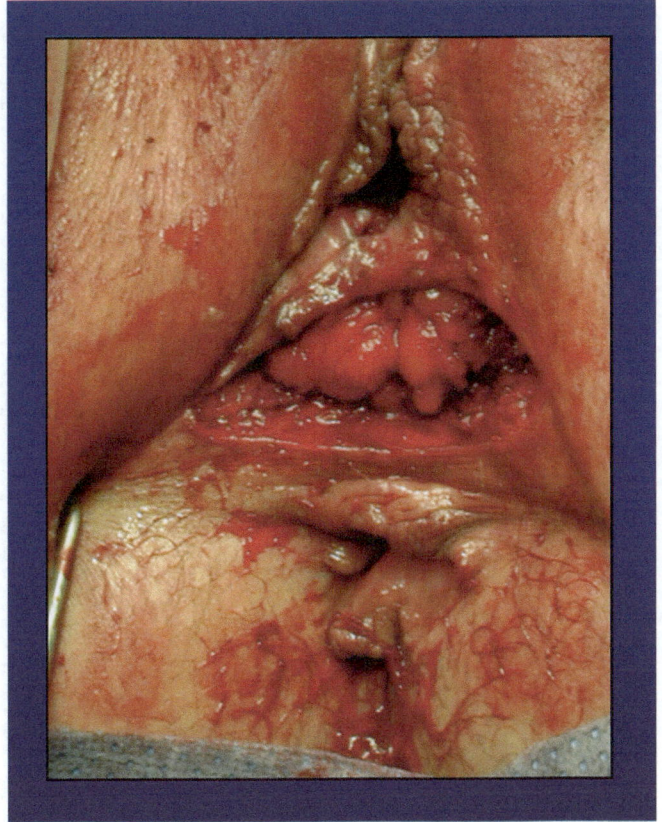

Fig. 16.6 The flap is located in its place

Warning Signs for Complications

Early warning signs of complications include increasing pain, urinary retention, and fever. These may be suggestive of a postoperative abscess. Early drainage from the fistula site is not necessarily a complication in the early postoperative period since many or most patients will continue to experience some drainage until the fistula is completely healed.

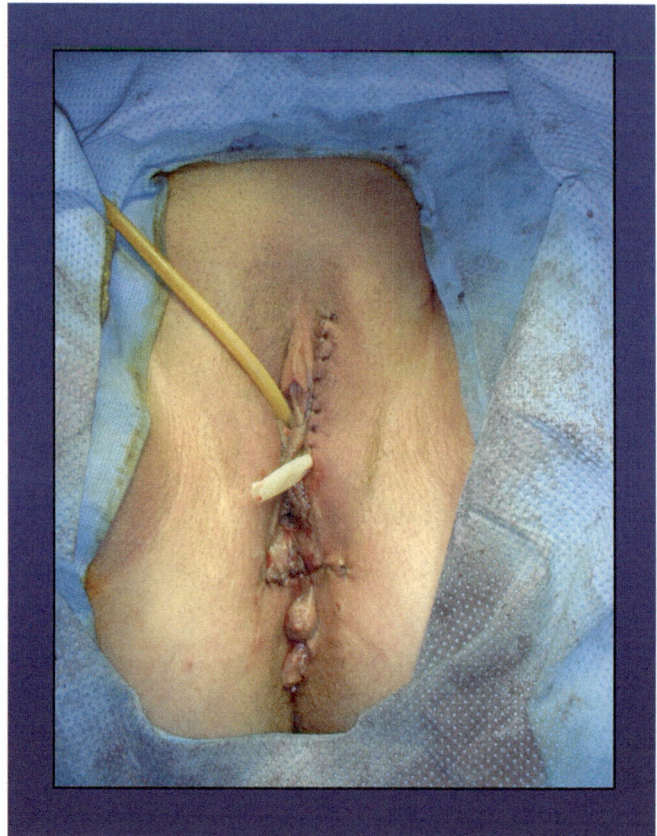

Fig. 16.7 Closure of all incisions

Clinical Pearls

As with many clinical problems, there are a variety of therapeutic choices for RVF. The treatment chosen must be individualized to the specific patient depending on anatomy, radiation history, obstetric history, and other underlying conditions. A typical fistula due to an obstetric injury can best be managed with sphinctero-plasty and flap. A flap can also manage most cryptoglandular fistulas. Thorough evaluation of anorectal function, obstetric history, and medical history is critical to help make the best choice for the planned operation. Newer techniques include the addition of a biologic or prosthetic mesh placed in the rectovaginal septum. At present, more data are required prior to our recommendations regarding these techniques.

Chapter 17
Ileoanal Anastomosis

Yehuda Kariv and Eli D. Ehrenpreis

Description of the Procedure

Ileoanal pouch anastomosis is frequently performed in patients who require total proctocolectomy (see Fig. 17.1). Performance of an ileoanal anastomosis allows for the avoidance of a permanent ileostomy and restores fecal continence. A straight ileoanal anastomosis has been successfully performed in some children with refractory ulcerative colitis (UC) with reasonable functional outcomes. However, in adults, the functional results of direct ileoanal anastomosis are not satisfactory with increased stool frequency and impaired continence. Therefore, current ileoanal anastomosis procedures usually involve creation of an ileal pouch as a "neorectum" with reservoir capacity. This procedure is called restorative proctocolectomy or ileal pouch–anal anastomosis (IPAA). In 1978, Parks and Nicholls described an ileal pouch reservoir in an S configuration that was handsewn to the anus following distal rectal mucosectomy. The S pouch was characterized by a long efferent limb that was associated with impaired pouch emptying and a suboptimal functional outcome. There followed a decade of experimentation with various pouch configurations, S, J, H and W, before the J configuration was accepted as the standard operative technique because of ease of construction and efficiency of evacuation. IPAA procedures originally involved mucosectomy, or excision of transitional mucosa above the dentate line, and a

Y. Kariv, MD (✉)
Tel Aviv Sourasky Medical Center, Colo-rectal Surgery Unit, Division of Surgery,
10 Weizman Street, Tel Aviv, Israel
e-mail: kariv_y@yahoo.com

E.D. Ehrenpreis, MD (✉)
Chief of Gastroenterology and Endoscopy, Highland Park Hospital,
NorthShore University Health System, Highland Park, IL 60035, USA

Clinical Associate Professor of Medicine, University of Chicago Medical Center,
Highland Park, IL 60035, USA
e-mail: ehrenpreis@gipharm.net

E.D. Ehrenpreis et al. (eds.), *Anal and Rectal Diseases: A Concise Manual*,
DOI 10.1007/978-1-4614-1102-4_17, © Springer Science+Business Media, LLC 2012

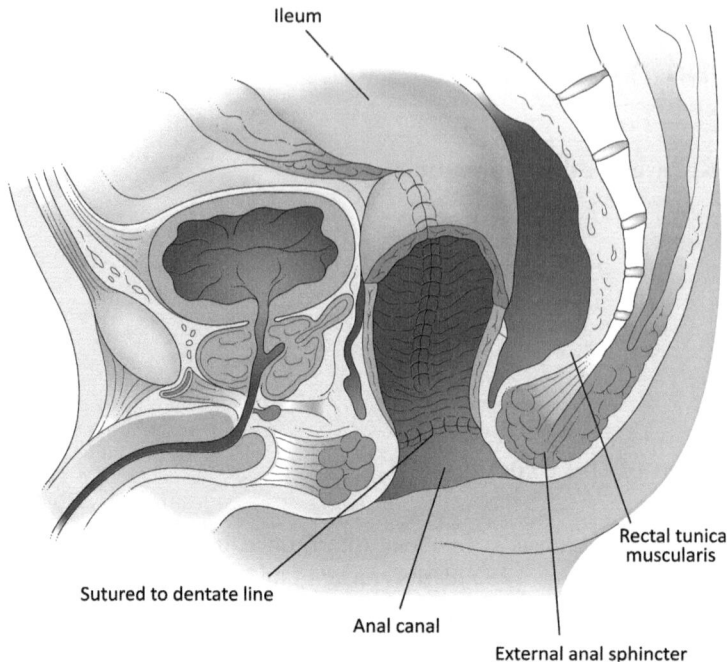

Ileum

Rectal tunica
muscularis

Sutured to dentate line

Anal canal

External anal sphincter

Fig. 17.1 Diagram of the ileoanal pouch anastomosis

handsewn anastomosis. Later, a double-stapled technique was developed, where 1–2 cm of the anal transitional zone mucosa above the dentate line is preserved with anastomosis to the proximal portion of the anal canal. The relative ease and speed of stapled IPAA has led to its widespread application. With these technical modifications, IPAA has evolved into the surgical treatment of choice for most patients with refractory UC or familial adenomatous polyposis (FAP).

Indications

The two most common indications for the IPAA are UC and FAP (see Table 17.1). IPAA has also been performed in selected patients with Crohn's disease, severe constipation due to colonic and rectal inertia, and Hirschsprung's disease. Up to 40% of patients with UC will eventually require surgery. Indications for surgery in UC patients include colitis refractory to medical management, steroid-dependent colitis, complications of medical management, severe or toxic colitis with or without megacolon, intractable bleeding, dysplasia or established colorectal cancer, and growth retardation in children or adolescents. Surgery to remove the colon and rectum is indicated in patients with FAP because all patients are at risk to develop colorectal cancer by the age of 40 unless a proctocolectomy is performed. In these patients, surgery is usually performed before the age of 20. Crohn's disease is generally

Table 17.1 Indications and contraindications for ileoanal pouch anastomosis

Indications	Contraindications	Relative contraindications
Chronic UC	Crohn's disease	Massive obesity
FAP	Cancer of the distal rectum	Emergency operation
Multiple colorectal malignancies	Poor anal sphincter function	Use of steroid medication
	Anal sphincter excised	Indeterminate colitis
	Age > 65 years	

considered a contraindication to IPAA owing to increased postoperative complications and long-term pouch failure. Pouch loss may be expected in up to 33% in those patients with postoperative recrudescent Crohn's disease. However, up to 90% of well-selected patients with a preoperative diagnosis of Crohn's disease may retain their pouch in the absence of preexisting ileal or perianal disease. The IPAA is usually successful in patients with indeterminate colitis but approximately 30% will manifest signs and symptoms of Crohn's disease within 10 years of the operation.

Contraindications

Absolute contraindications to performance of an IPAA procedure include carcinoma in the low rectum requiring a total anorectal excision and an incompetent anal sphincter (Table 17.1). Patients with UC presenting as an emergency should be treated with a colectomy and ileostomy with preservation of the rectum. A period of at least 3 months should elapse before undertaking completion proctectomy and construction of an IPAA.

Relative Contraindications

Crohn's disease is a relative contraindication for an IPAA procedure. Primary sclerosing cholangitis may increase pouchitis and ileal pouch dysplasia rates in patients with UC after an IPAA procedure, and these risks should be discussed with the patient prior to surgery. Restorative proctocolectomy may decrease fertility rate in women of child-bearing age. The options include accepting the risk of reduced fertility with a restorative proctocolectomy or having a colectomy and ileostomy to treat the disease followed by restorative proctocolectomy at the patient's convenience after having children. IPAA was initially reserved for younger patients, but following an overall decrease in morbidity rates the operation has become a more attractive option for the older age group. Studies reported that the procedure was safe and feasible, and yielded good functional results, in patients over 50 years of age. The overall functional outcome of IPAA in patients over 65 years of age is satisfactory, and the procedure is a realistic choice for continence preservation even in selected patients in their eighth decade.

Alternatives

About two-thirds of patients with UC are successfully managed with medications and do not require surgery during their lifetime. Medical management of UC includes aminosalicylates, steroids, immunomodulating agents, biologic therapy, and others. When surgery is indicated in UC patients, an IPAA procedure is most common surgery performed. Alternative surgical procedures in UC patients include conventional proctocolectomy and ileostomy, and colectomy with ileorectal anastomosis. The last of these is only suitable for the few patients whose rectum is relatively free of inflammation and where there is no dysplasia or established cancer in the large bowel. Colectomy with ileorectal anastomosis is also an alternative in patients with attenuated FAP (less than 100 colonic polyps and limited rectal involvement) and well-selected classic FAP patients with limited rectal disease. Careful endoscopic surveillance of the remaining rectum is required in these patients. The continent ileostomy of Kock (known as the Kock pouch) is an alternative to a conventional end ileostomy in patients who require total proctocolectomy and are not good candidates for IPAA (e.g., poor sphincter tone), or those in whom an IPAA has failed. It involves the creation of an ileal reservoir with a nipple valve. It has not enjoyed widespread acceptance because of relatively high risk of pouch dysfunction.

How the Procedure Is Performed

Restorative proctocolectomy involves removal of the colon and rectum and construction of a reservoir or "pouch" from the last 30–40 cm of ileum followed by an ileoanal anastomosis. Usually, the rectum is transected at the level of the levator ani muscles or the anorectal junction. Most surgeons use a J- or two-loop pouch configuration owing to the ease of construction. The J-shaped pouch is constructed by stapling two 15–20 cm limbs of ileum together with a gastrointestinal anastomosis (linear stapler) (GIA) anastomotic staler. In forming the IPAA, the surgeon can either staple or handsew the pouch to the anal canal. This is an important consideration because stapling leaves a 1–2-cm cuff of residual rectal mucosa in situ, which may become symptomatic and is at risk of dysplasia. The handsewn technique includes a mucosectomy to remove virtually all rectal mucosa above the dentate line and places the anastomosis just at the dentate line, but it may be associated with a higher incidence of minor anal leakage. Controversy remains concerning the indications for mucosectomy. Today, a majority of IPAA procedures involves a stapled anastomosis. A stapled anastomosis is performed using a end to end anastomosis (circular stapler) (EEA) transanal stapler.

Total proctocolectomy and IPAA can be performed in either one, two or three stages. A three stage operation is usually undertaken in acutely unwell patients with UC when subtotal colectomy with end ileostomy and preservation of the rectal stump is performed as the first stage. Completion proctectomy and IPAA with a diverting loop ileostomy is undertaken following an interval of at least 3 months. Closure of the ileostomy is usually performed at least 8 weeks after the second

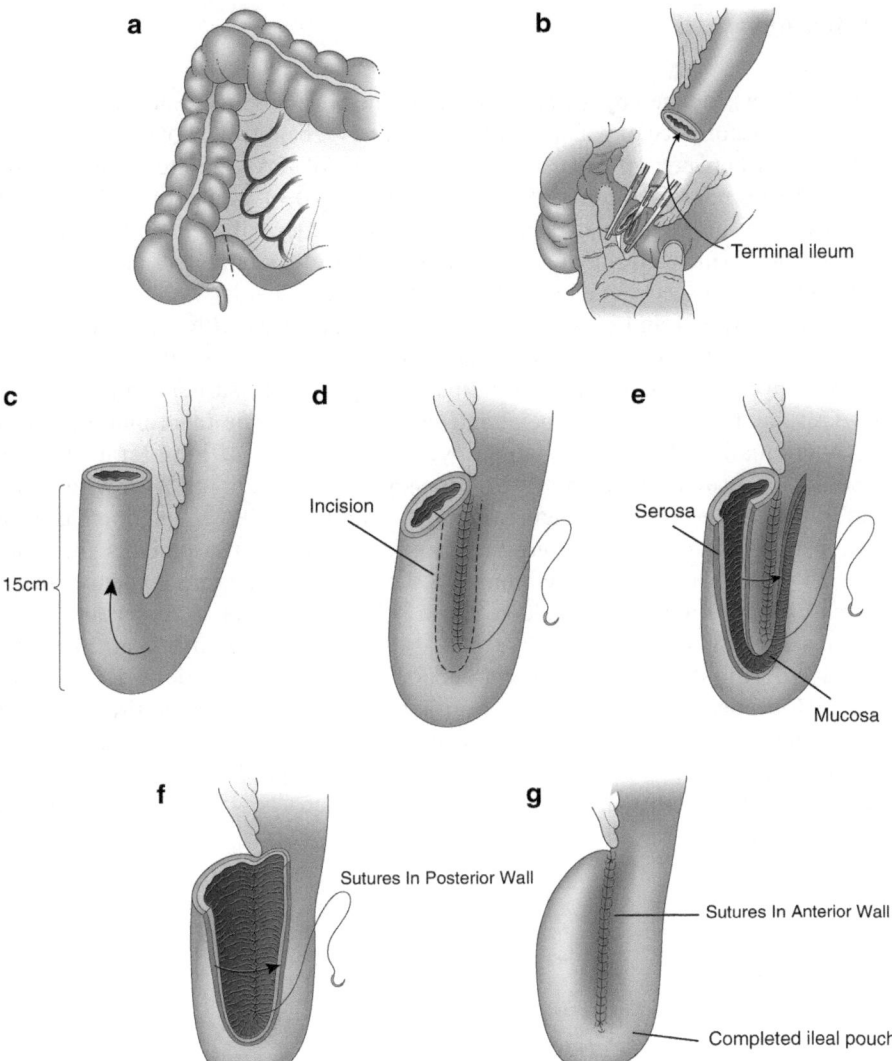

Fig. 17.2 Construction of a handsewn j shaped ileal pouch. (**a, b**) The terminal ileum is divided and the colon is removed. (**c**) The terminal ileum is fashioned into a J-shape with 15 cm limbs. (**d, e**) The antimesenteric border of the ileum is divided. (**f**) The posterior wall of the pouch is sutured. (**g**) The pouch is completed

stage. In systemically well patients, restorative proctocolectomy is usually undertaken in two stages: (1) total proctocolectomy, IPAA, and loop ileostomy, and (2) closure of loop ileostomy. However, some surgeons use a one-stage technique to avoid a defunctioning ileostomy.

An IPAA procedure can be performed using minimally invasive approaches (e.g., laparoscopy, hand-assisted laparoscopy). A minimally invasive approach might have short-term benefits and better cosmetic results (see Fig. 17.2).

Outcomes

Pouch failure is defined by the need to remove the pouch or indefinitely establish an ileostomy. Occurrence of pouch failure is cumulative, being about 5% at 5 years and 8–15% after between 10 and 20 years. The causes of IPAA failure include pelvic sepsis (50%), poor function (30%), and pouchitis (10%). Approximately 25% of failures occur during the first year. Surgical revision after failure of an IPAA is possible in some patients through a perineal or combined abdominoperineal approach and may yield an acceptable level of bowel function.

Most functional and quality of life data related to the IPAA originate from series of patients with UC. Functional results and quality of life after surgery improve over time such that approximately 1 year after surgery most patients have resumed normal work, social and sexual activity. The favorable impact of IPAA on quality of life is sustained over time. Reports of long-term function have demonstrated a median stool frequency of 4–8 stools per 24 h with about half of patients needing to evacuate at night. Stability of IPAA function has been demonstrated to occur in a long-term study that monitored patients for more than 25 years. Urgency is uncommon, although there is some evidence that it increases with time. Fecal leakage during the day occurs in less than 4% of patients. At night, these rates are 4% at 10 years rising to 9% at 25 years. Seepage during the day and at night occurs in 7 and 9% of patients rising to 11 and 18%, respectively, at 25 years. Antidiarrhea medication is required in about a third of patients at 10 years and 45% at 25 years. Overall, the vast majority of patients report their result as satisfactory. The IPAA produces a greater overall improvement in quality of life than either an end ileostomy or Kock pouch (continent ileostomy).

Complications

Anastomotic Leak (Pelvic Sepsis)

IPAA has a low operative mortality (0.4%), but is associated with an early morbidity rate of approximately 30%. The most important complication in the early postoperative period is breakdown of the ileoanal anastomosis (anastomotic leak) with consequent pelvic sepsis (see Fig. 17.3). This occurs in 5–10% of patients and is associated with a fivefold risk of long-term failure. Some cases will resolve with antibiotic treatment only, and others require surgical drainage. If not already present, a defunctioning ileostomy may be required.

Fig. 17.3 Ileoanal pouch anastomosis. Several small anastomotic leaks are demonstrated on dynamic proctography (*arrow*)

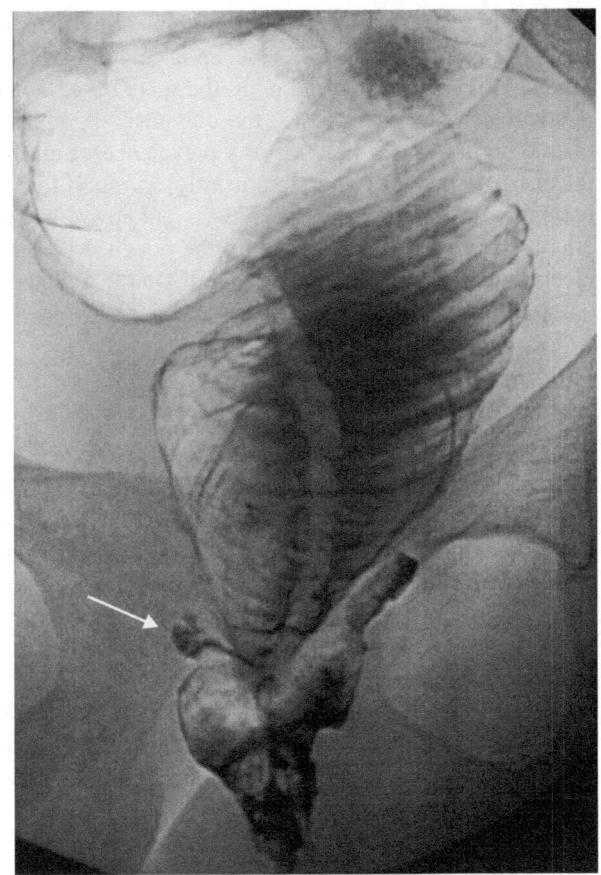

Fistulization

Fistulization from the pouch to the vagina or the perineum can occur any time following surgery with an incidence of 5–10% over 10 years. The main risk factors include pelvic sepsis in the early postoperative period, indeterminate colitis, and Crohn's disease unrecognized at the time of IPAA procedure.

Pouchitis

Some degree of pouch inflammation in the ileal pouch ("pouchitis") develops in up to 50% of patients with UC after restorative proctocolectomy. Pouchitis is much less frequent in FAP patients. Pouchitis is diagnosed when histologically proven acute inflammation is associated with symptoms of frequency, urgency, and liquid stool in the presence of endoscopic evidence of inflammation. The high quoted incidences of pouchitis may be misleading as these are based on cumulative life table analysis methodology. In many cases, the diagnosis of pouchitis was not confirmed with histology. In clinical practice, the prevalence of chronic persisting pouchitis (and thus of patients suffering significantly) is much lower, occurring in about 5% of patients. The etiology of pouchitis is unknown, but is likely to be related to the alteration in bacterial flora within the pouch. Mucosal edema, granularity, and/or ulcerations may be seen endoscopically in the affected pouch.

Chronic Pouchitis

A small percentage of patients develop recurrent or chronic pouchitis, and half of these patients will need resection of the pouch. The standard treatment is metronidazole (10–20 mg/kg/day), sometimes in combination with ciprofloxacin (500 mg b.i.d.). Treatment duration is usually 2–4 weeks. Chronic pouchitis has been treated with 5-acetylsalicylic acid (5-ASA), containing agents such as Pentasa or mesalamine enemas, and immunosuppressant drugs (i.e., corticosteroids, azathioprine, short-chain fatty acid enemas, and probiotics). Administration of live probiotic bacteria has been demonstrated to maintain remission in patients with chronic pouchitis. Only 10% of pouch failures are due to the development of pouchitis. Other complications include early and late bowel obstruction, anastomostic strictures, pouch ulcers (see Fig. 17.4), and stomal complications; furthermore, an impotence rate of 3.8% has been reported.

Dysplasia and Cancer

Depending on the type of rectal dissection performed, a small portion of the rectal mucosa from the anal transition zone can be left at the site of the anastomosis. This cuff of rectal tissue is larger when (without than) a double-stapled technique is used. Although rare, dysplasia and carcinoma have been reported in this remaining portion of rectal mucosa. Current recommendations include surveillance sigmoidoscopy with biopsy at the site of anastomosis every 1–3 years.

Warning Signs for Complications

Patients should be monitored for postoperative bleeding. Ileus, fever, purulent anal discharge, anal pain, and abdominal tenderness may signify septic complications. Abdominal pain and vomiting may also be manifestations of bowel obstruction. Diarrhea and pelvic pain suggest the presence of pouchitis. Patients should be monitored for long-term complications including pouchitis, fecal leakage, and impotence.

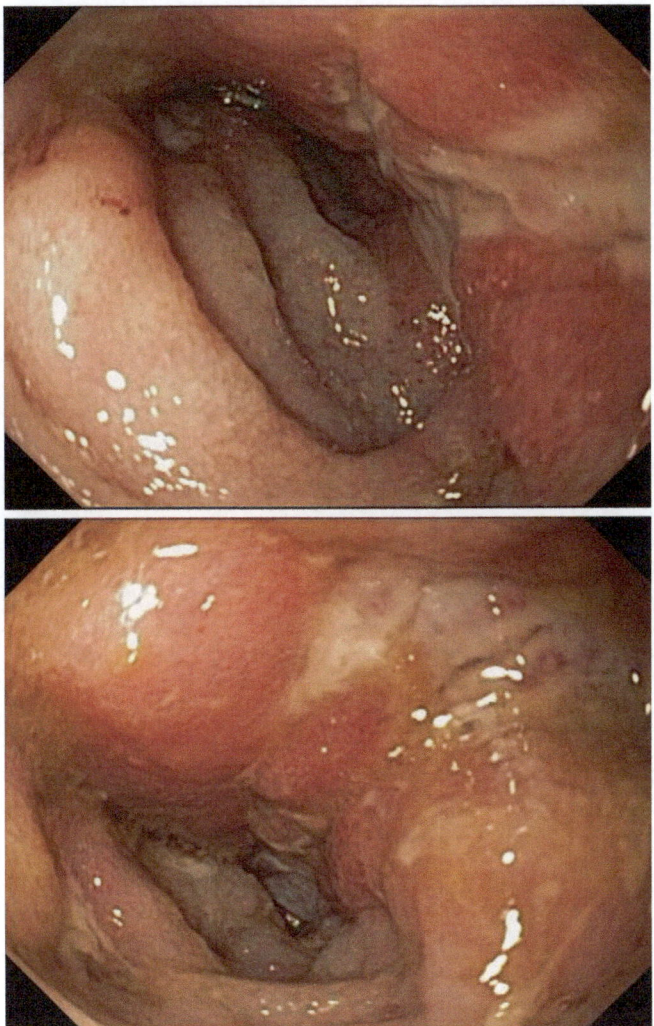

Fig. 17.4 Endoscopic view of a large superficial ulceration seen at the anastomosis of the J-pouch and ileum. Biopsies were suggestive of Crohn's disease of the pouch and small bowel

Routine periodic follow-up with pouch endoscopy is required in both UC and FAP patients for early detection of dysplasia and cancer.

Clinical Pearls

The IPAA is a challenging operation to perform. Patient outcomes after IPAA have been shown to be better in institutions with higher volumes of procedures compared to those who perform the procedure infrequently. IPAA can be constructed either through a laparotomy incision or using a minimally invasive approach. Despite its association with significant morbidity, pouch survival and good functional results are reported in the majority of cases. Careful selection of the specific surgical procedure in patients with UC and FAP is mandatory to decrease short-term and long-term complication rates, and to optimize functional results and quality of life.

Chapter 18
Bowel Reconstruction Following Low Anterior Resection

Shmuel Avital

Background

A low anterior resection using the total mesorectal excision (TME) approach is usually performed for low and mid rectal tumors. Patients may suffer from evacuation difficulties following a low anterior resection generally called post anterior resection syndrome. This syndrome is more evident following a straight coloanal anastomosis (SCA) (Fig. 18.1a) and has been reported in up to 60% of patients.

Post anterior resection syndrome involves frequent bowel movements, fecal and gas leakage, urgency, and difficulty emptying that leads to an impaired quality of life. Pelvic irradiation and low pelvic anastomosis after rectal resection have been demonstrated to negatively affect bowel function. The development of post anterior resection syndrome is related to an impairment of the anorectal reflex, which is the transient relaxation of the internal anal sphincter in response to rectal balloon dilation, decreased motor function of the neorectum, and removal of the rectal reservoir. However, there is a gradual improvement in these symptoms over a 2-year period following surgery.

Several surgical approaches for neorectal reconstruction have been offered to improve the symptoms associated with post anterior resection syndrome. Using the left colon instead of the sigmoid colon may be superior as it is more pliable and may serve as a better reservoir.

S. Avital, MD (✉)
Chief of Surgery, Department of Surgery B, Meir Medical Center, Kfar-Saba, Israel
e-mail: avitalshmuel@gmail.com

E.D. Ehrenpreis et al. (eds.), *Anal and Rectal Diseases: A Concise Manual*,
DOI 10.1007/978-1-4614-1102-4_18, © Springer Science+Business Media, LLC 2012

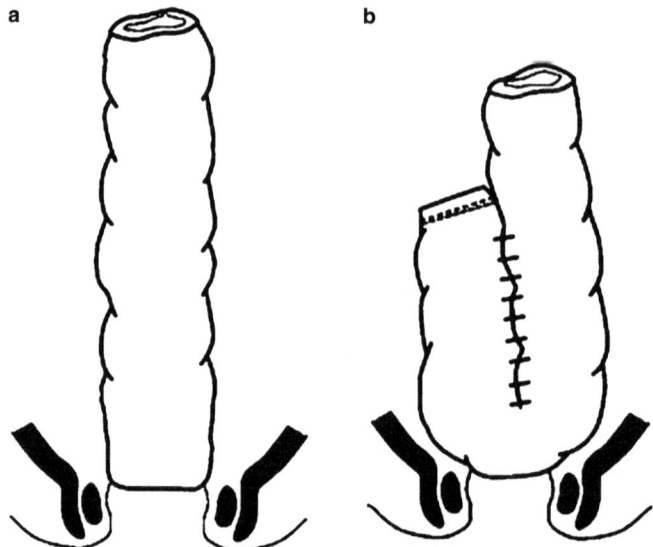

Fig. 18.1 (a) SCA. (b) CJP anal anastomosis

Procedures

There are three procedures for neorectal reconstruction that were reported to achieve improved functional results compared to a SCA. These procedures include the following:

1. Transverse coloplasty (TC)
2. Colonic J pouch (CJP) creation
3. Side-to-end (STE) anastomosis with a blind loop

   The first two methods are generally protected by a diverting ileostomy.

General Description/Goals of Surgery

How the Surgery Is Performed

Transverse Coloplasty

A longitudinal incision, about 8 cm in length, is performed from 2 cm proximal to the end of the colon that is going to be anastomosed to the distal rectal stump. The incision is then closed transversely with sutures. An anastomosis is then created to the colonic end (Fig. 18.2).

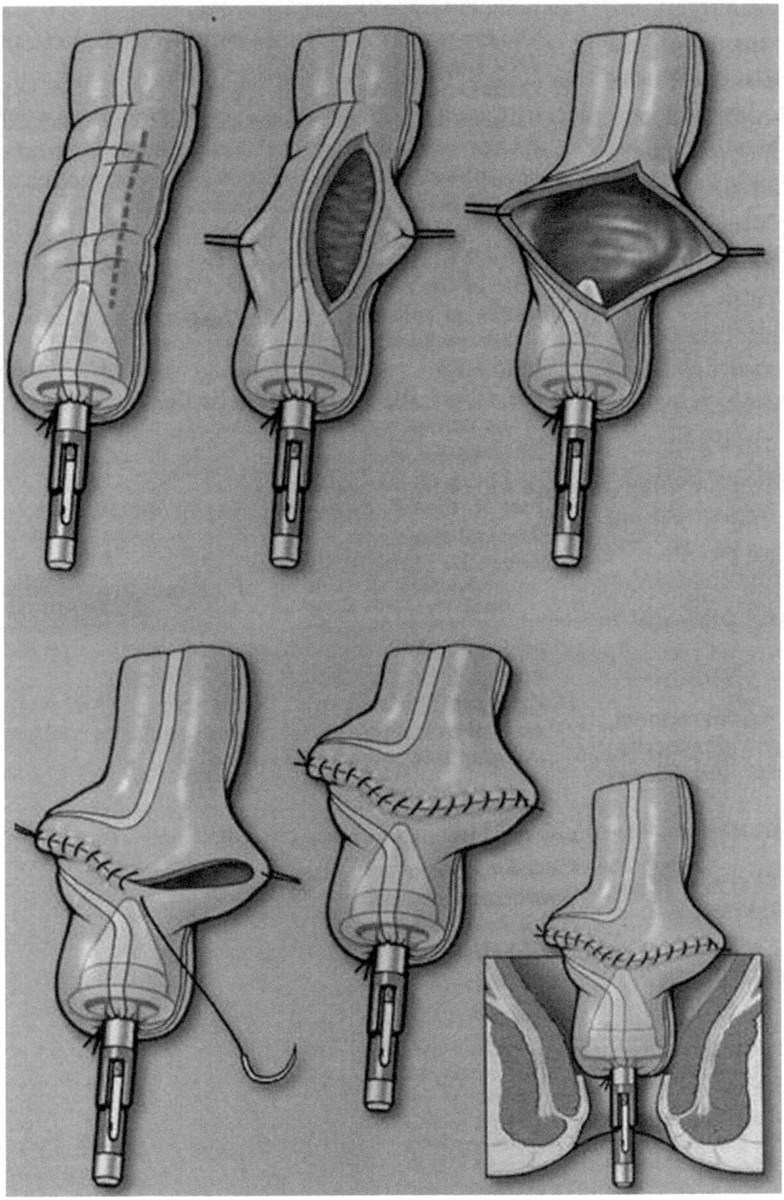

Fig. 18.2 Surgical technique of the TC pouch (end-to-end anastomosis)

Colonic J Pouch

This procedure is similar to the ileal pouch anal anastomosis performed after proctocolectomy for ulcerative colitis or familial adenomatous polyposis (FAP). A limb of the sigmoid or, preferably, the left colon is folded on itself in a J fashion to serve as the neorectal reservoir. The end of this segment should be sutured closed. The pouch is created by attaching the two arms of the J through an opening on its J tip and then firing a 6–8-cm linear stapler. The anastomosis is then performed with a circular stapler from the anal canal/distal rectal stump to the tip of the J pouch (Fig. 18.1b).

When creating a J pouch, it is necessary to mobilize the splenic flexure and to perform a high ligation of the inferior mesenteric artery and transecting the inferior mesenteric vein in order that the left colon J limb can reach the low pelvis.

Side-To-End Anastomosis with a Blind Loop

This last procedure is, surgically, the easiest to perform. This procedure entails creating a reservoir by simply anastomosing the side tip of a J limb to the distal rectal stump or anal canal and leaving a 5-cm blind J arm without constructing a pouch. In this way, a neorectal reservoir is created.

Contraindications

Patients with anal incontinence should not have an anastomosis, in which case a permanent stoma should be created.

Indications

Patients who undergo low anterior resection with sphincter preservation and who have reasonable anal continence prior to surgery.

Relative Contraindications

Obese patients, in particular male patients with a narrow pelvis, are not good candidates for a J pouch as they not have enough length of colon and it may not be possible to reconstruct the colon within the pelvis.

Alternatives

The alternative to reconstruction of a neorectum is the creation of a permanent stoma.

Outcomes

1. Studies comparing J pouch vs. SCA have shown improvement in evacuation impairment up to 2 years following surgery. The CJP was superior to SCA in most studies in bowel frequency, urgency, anal incontinence, and the use of antidiarrheal medications. Two years after surgery, this difference was diminishing due to gradual improvement in the function of the SCA.
2. Studies comparing STE anastomosis to the CJP showed no difference in bowel function outcome between these two techniques. Similarly, several small studies comparing TC to CJP demonstrated no differences in bowel function outcome between these groups.
3. Overall, there were no significant differences in postoperative complications with any of the anastomotic strategies. However, the data are still limited.

Complications

Early

The most significant early complication is anastomotic leak. The risk for anastomotic leak increases in very low anastomoses and in irradiated patients. As a rule, it is recommended to construct a diverting loop ileostomy to lower the rate of significant leaks and pelvic sepsis. This is recommended in irradiated patients and following TC and CJP. In cases of STE anastomosis and no irradiation, avoiding the need of an ileostomy may be considered.

Late

All other complications are related to the low anterior resection and are detailed in the surgical section on rectal cancer.

Warning Signs for Complications

Pelvic leaks do not necessarily cause peritonitis. Patients who may be at risk for pelvic leaks develop fever, malaise, distended abdomen and ileus, and tenesmus. Fecal discharge may be noted from drains that are left in the pelvis and should alert to possible pelvic leak.

Clinical Pearls

1. Post anterior resection syndrome impairs quality of life following low anterior resection.
2. There are currently three methods of anastomotic reconstruction to improve functional outcome following anterior resection.
3. The most studied method is CJP. It was been shown to lead to better bowel function and a similar complication rate compared to SCA.
4. The improved bowel function following CJP seems to persist up to 2 years and thereafter, which is similar to SCA.
5. There is more limited data on with the TC and STE techniques; however, these data demonstrate similar functional results for all three techniques.
6. There is some evidence that TC may result in a higher rate of anastomotic leak.
7. If STE anastomosis consistently proves to be as good as SCA or CJP, it may be preferred because of its ease of reconstruction, especially in obese and male patients.

Chapter 19
Transanal Resection of Rectal Lesions

Shmuel Avital

Description of Procedures

There are two common techniques for transanal excision of anorectal lesions. Conventional transanal excision involves operation through the anal canal. Lesions that are more proximal, and therefore difficult to visualize and reach with conventional instrumentation, may be better suited for transanal endoscopic microsurgery (TEM).

Indications

Indications include benign polyps and early rectal cancers. Polyps are thoroughly investigated prior to embarking on transanal resection. Assessment may include biopsy, endoscopic ultrasound (EUS), CT or MRI, and/or serum tumor markers. The decision to perform a transanal excision is independent of the technical aspects (in other words, whether to perform a transanal excision or TEM). If the anorectal lesion is found to be malignant on evaluation, staging is required (using EUS or MRI) so that neoadjuvant chemoradiation can be performed in appropriate patients. Most surgeons would agree that T1 rectal tumors may be potentially suitable for transanal excision, while T2 lesions are only safe to excise transanally under highly selected circumstances. T3, T4, or node-positive disease should not be resected transanally for cure. Patients unfit for radical resection (low anterior resection [LAR] or abdominoperineal resection [APR]), may be managed with local excision, but this should not be reliably offered as a curative procedure in patients with more advanced disease.

S. Avital, MD (✉)
Chief of Surgery, Department of Surgery B, Meir Medical Center, Kfar-Saba, Israel
e-mail: avitalshmuel@gmail.com

E.D. Ehrenpreis et al. (eds.), *Anal and Rectal Diseases: A Concise Manual*,
DOI 10.1007/978-1-4614-1102-4_19, © Springer Science+Business Media, LLC 2012

Contraindications

Patients who are unable to undergo anesthesia (see Chap. 24).

Relative Contraindications

Relative contraindications include patients with metastatic disease. The management of patients with metastatic rectal cancer is evolving. There is discussion on the necessity of resection of the primary tumor while treating metastatic rectal cancer. However, if the primary tumor is symptomatic (i.e., bleeding), then excision is indicated. These patients will require an APR, unless excision is being performed as a palliative measure only.

Alternatives

The alternatives to transanal excision include radical resection (LAR or APR), endoscopic removal, or nonoperative treatment such as chemoradiation.

How the Operation Is Performed

Transanal excision is usually an outpatient procedure. Conventional transanal excision is performed in the operating room. General, regional, or local anesthesia may be employed at the discretion of the patient and surgeon, and according to the location of the tumor. Exposure of the perineum is best while patents are in the prone jack-knife position; however, the lithotomy position may facilitate excision of posterior lesions. If regional or general anesthesia is used, local anesthetics should also be infiltrated into the sphincter to allow for maximal dilation and best exposure of the lesion. Lesions in the anal canal or distal rectum can typically be visualized with conventional anoscopy with a Hill-Ferguson or similar instrument. Local anesthetic with epinephrine should be infiltrated at the base of the lesion to control bleeding. If a partial thickness excision is planned for benign lesions, injection of saline into the submucosa will provide hydrodissection and improve hemostasis. The lesion should then be grasped and excised by sharp dissection or cautery. If the lesion is larger, then it may be helpful to place a suture into the tumor to provide traction. The planned excision should be mapped by scoring the mucosa with cautery. The dissection should be started at the distal aspect of the lesion, where it is best visualized. The dissection should be carried from distal to proximal. If a full-thickness excision is planned, the borders of the lesion should definitely be scored. Stay sutures should be placed into the specimen. Lesions in the infraperitoneal rectum or anus do not necessarily require closure, as these will heal on their own. Proximal lesions, especially in the anterior rectum, should be closed. This can be performed with simple interrupted or running sutures. The defects should be closed transversely to avoid narrowing of the lumen. Sometimes, this may require alternative equipment such as the Lone Star retractor or an operating proctoscope.

TEM requires special equipment. This consists of a specifically designed operating proctoscope. It is 40 mm in diameter. There is a specific faceplate that allows for the introduction of the optics system as well as operating instruments. The rectum is insufflated with air to distend the bowel and allow for visualization of abnormalities. A camera is inserted so that the surgeon may work from the video monitors with the aid of magnification, similar to laparoscopy. There are two or three working channels that allow for the introduction of graspers, scissors, cautery, suction, or needle drivers. The lesion is visualized, and a needle tipped cautery instrument is used to map the excision by scoring out the planned excision along with a margin of normal tissue. An epinephrine-containing solution can be infiltrated into the submucosa if a partial thickness excision is planned. The lesion is grasped with one instrument, and a cautery or energy device (such as Harmonic) is used to perform the excision. The excision is performed in the bimucosal plane for partial thickness excisions, or all the way through the rectal wall for full thickness excisions. Once the lesion is fully mobilized, it is removed through the proctoscope. The defect can be left open if it is a partial thickness removal. If the wound is going to be closed, an absorbable suture is placed into the apex of the defect. A silver bead is placed at the beginning of the suture to anchor it in place. This avoids the need to tie knots, which can be cumbersome. Full thickness closure of the defect is performed in a transverse direction. Another silver bead is applied at the completion of the closure avoiding the need for tying of sutures.

Outcomes

Outcomes depend primarily on the indication for excision. The procedure is generally well tolerated. If the lesion is very distal, sutures may be near the dentate line and can therefore cause pain. This may require hospitalization for pain control. The most significant possible complication of transanal excision is the recurrence of the excised lesion. Patients should undergo postoperative surveillance with endoscopy at regular intervals to monitor for recurrence. Recurrence rates of early stage rectal cancers are the primary outcome of concern regarding local excision techniques. It is unclear whether these recurrences represent an inadequate excision, or nodal recurrence of microscopic disease. Unlike local excisions, radical excision properly stages the initial tumor and possibly results in the removal of malignant mesorectal nodes. Recurrence rates after transanal resection have been reported up to 23% tor T1 lesions (compared to 6% for surgical excision). The recurrence rate for radical vs. transanal resection of low-risk lesions (upper or middle rectal tumors with low to moderate differentiation, without evidence of local lymphatic invasion) is low and may be similar for both approaches (0–5%).

Complications

Early complications for both techniques include bleeding, pain, abscess formation, and urinary retention. Late complications include tumor recurrence, or sphincter injury from dilation. The 40 mm proctoscope is large, but generally accommodated with sufficient relaxation of the sphincter. Although not previously reported, dilation could potentially cause a stretch injury resulting in fecal incontinence.

Warning Signs for Complications

The triad of fever, pain, and urinary retention can be concerning for the development of pelvic sepsis. This triad of symptoms should prompt immediate return to the office or hospital.

Clinical Pearls

The most important decisions regarding transanal excision involve the indication for the procedure. There is no question that benign lesions, particularly adenomatous polyps can be safely excised transanally. Since these are benign mucosal lesions, partial thickness excision is indicated. For rectal cancers, the issue is more controversial. Patients should have full disclosure of published recurrence rates so they can make an informed decision about removal of these lesions by the transanal route. There is no question that short-term outcomes and postoperative morbidity are dramatically better than radical resections, but patients must understand the tradeoff of potentially increased recurrence rates with local excision.

Chapter 20
Laparoscopic Rectal Resection

Shmuel Avital

Introduction

Several large, prospective, randomized studies have demonstrated benefits from the use of laparoscopic surgery for colon cancer compared to open laparotomy. Laparoscopic colon cancer surgery is associated with a shorter and easier postoperative recovery. These advantages have also been shown for rectosigmoid cancers including upper rectal tumors (12–18 cm from the anal verge). However, there are very few prospective randomized trials evaluating the oncologic safety and benefits of laparoscopic resection for cancer in the lower two-thirds of the rectum.

Unlike laparoscopic surgery in the colon, the anatomy of the rectum – which is confined to the narrow bony pelvis and attached anteriorly to the vagina in women and seminal vesicles and prostate in males – makes laparoscopic surgery in this region very challenging.

Because of these considerations, the role of laparoscopy as a surgical modality in rectal cancer is still debated, and this procedure is primarily being practiced by dedicated laparoscopic colorectal surgeons or is confined to clinical trials.

Procedure

Laparoscopic procedures performed for rectal cancer include anterior resection or abdominoperineal resection (APR). These procedures are performed based on the currently accepted oncologic approach of total mesorectal excision (TME). TME includes complete excision of the mesorectum using sharp dissection via distinct

S. Avital, MD (✉)
Chief of Surgery, Department of Surgery B, Meir Medical Center, Kfar-Saba, Israel
e-mail: avitalshmuel@gmail.com

E.D. Ehrenpreis et al. (eds.), *Anal and Rectal Diseases: A Concise Manual*,
DOI 10.1007/978-1-4614-1102-4_20, © Springer Science+Business Media, LLC 2012

anatomical planes with sparing of autonomic genitourinary nerves. The performance of these two procedures is identical to their open method counterparts, as described in complete detail in Chap. 21.

General Description/Goals of Surgery

The aim of this surgery is to completely remove the rectum, including the mesorectum, and achieve clear histological margins. Reconstruction with anastomosis of the proximal colon to the distal rectal stump or anal canal is the second goal. The principles of each procedure are detailed in Chap. 21.

Indications

The main indication for laparoscopy in the anorectal region is rectal cancer. Other rare indications are laparoscopic APR for recurrent or persistent anal canal cancer following radiotherapy and chemotherapy, and laparoscopic rectal resection for rectal polyps that cannot be removed via the anus by local excision or transanal endoscopic microsurgery (TEM).

Contraindications

Locally advanced tumor, with penetration to adjacent organs including the prostate, vagina, or the sacrum are contraindications for laparoscopic resection.

Relative Contraindications

Relative contraindications include patients who are not candidates for extensive operations involving the production of a CO_2 pneumoperitoneum such as patients with chronic obstructive pulmonary disease (COPD) and/or congestive heart failure (CHF).

Alternatives

The main alternative – and currently still the method of choice – is an open surgical approach.

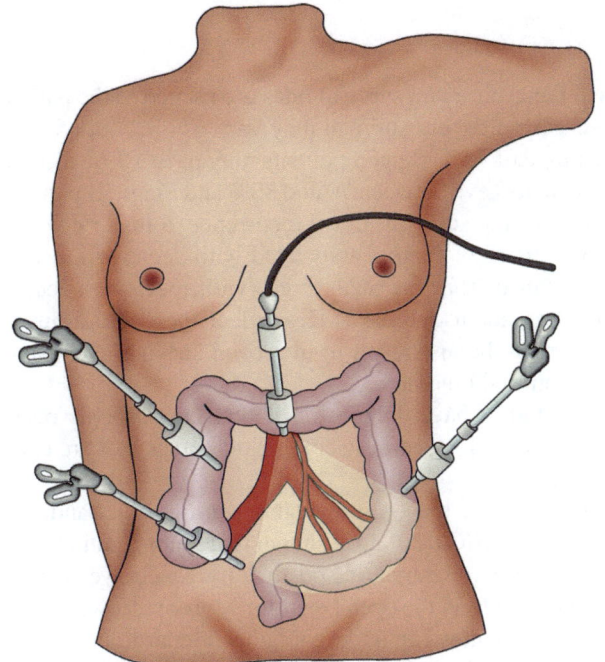

Fig. 20.1 Laparoscopic rectal surgery setup. Two trocars are localized at the lower part of the abdomen and one trocar at the right middle part. From SpringerImages: http://www.springerimages.com/Images/MedicineAndPublicHealth/1-10.1007_s00423-009-0556-y-0

How the Surgery Is Performed

The main principles for surgery for rectal cancer are described in Chap. 21. When performed laparoscopically, the abdominal cavity is insufflated with CO_2 up to a 15-mmHg pressure. A laparoscopic camera is inserted through a small incision, usually above the umbilicus (see Fig. 20.1). Three more small incisions are made, in which specific working instruments are inserted. Unlike the open approach, the dissection in laparoscopy is usually based on a medial-to-lateral approach. The first step is dissection of the inferior mesenteric artery (IMA) with its ligation, followed by a medial dissection of the mesorectum and mesosigmoid. Further, lateral dissection and a pelvic dissection are performed based on the TME principles. The next step is the distal rectal transection. This step is often difficult, given the limitation in angling of laparoscopic instruments. Following the distal transection, a small (5–6 cm) Pfannenstiel incision is made, and these transected mesorectum and mesosigmoid are exteriorized. A proximal transection is performed and the specimen is removed. The incision is sutured closed and the abdomen is reinsufflated. The anastomosis is performed laparoscopically, using a circular stapling device that is inserted through the anus.

Outcomes

Generally, local recurrence and survival rates are related to the pathological stage of the tumor. Disease-free 5-year survival may vary from about 65–70%, with overall survival in the range of 75%. Stage I patients may have 100% disease-free survival, while Stage II patients have between 70 and 80% and Stage III patients have between 50 and 60% disease-free survival. Local recurrence, a major concern in rectal cancer, ranges from 3 to 15%. Factors associated with decreased local recurrences are greater tumor distance from the anal verge (with the lowest local recurrence for upper rectal tumors), and use of the TME surgical approach. Adjuvant radiotherapy and neoadjuvant radiotherapy result in improved survival compared to no irradiation and no adjuvant radiotherapy.

Retrospective studies have demonstrated that laparoscopic resection for rectal cancer is safe and offers long-term oncologic outcomes that are equivalent to those of open resection.

However, results from the only available multicenter, randomized controlled study (UK MRC CLASSIC trial) have shown that among patients undergoing anterior resection, circumferential margins positive for cancer were found in 12% in the laparoscopic group vs. 6% in the open laparotomy group. However, improved cancer-free margins in the patient group undergoing open laparotomy did not translate into differences in 3-year local recurrence, disease-free survival, or overall survival. The findings from this study do warrant caution when determining the optimal surgical approach in a patient with rectal cancer.

Conversion to Open Laparotomy

Conversion to an open procedure is more common in laparoscopic rectal resection than in laparoscopic colon surgery, ranging from 5% to more than 30% of cases. Conversion to laparotomy has been associated with poorer short- and long-term patient outcomes. The negative impact of conversion may be a reflection of the factors that led to conversion to an open procedure, rather than the actual conversion itself.

Complications

The same complications that may occur following open resection can also arise after laparoscopic rectal resection.

Early Complications

Intraoperative Bleeding

Major bleeding may arise from the presacral venous complex when the posterior dissection is not accurate. This bleeding may be very difficult to control laparoscopically and may warrant conversion to an open procedure. Surgical management consists of packing and hemorrhage occluder pins (thumb tacks).

Anastomotic Leak

There is no evidence that the anastomotic leak rate is different between open laparotomy and laparoscopic surgery. Leak rates vary from 2 to 10%. Clinical manifestations of anastomotic leaks may vary from mild, controlled local infection to fulminant sepsis. Low anastomosis and neoadjuvant radiotherapy are associated with increased leak rates. Constructing a diverting loop ileostomy in the initial surgery is recommended in cases of very low anastomosis or following irradiation. Diverting ileostomy does not necessarily lower the anastomotic leak rate, but does decrease the occurrence of associated septic complications. When utilized, a diverting ileostomy is usually closed 6–12 weeks after surgery.

Wound Infection

Wound infections may develop in 10–20% of patients and can be managed with drainage and antibiotics, when necessary. Wound infections following laparoscopic rectal surgery (vs. an open procedure) are less significant, since the incisions are much smaller.

Unhealed perineal wounds following laparoscopic APR may occur in up to 25% of patients. Some of these may require surgical intervention.

Late Complications

Impaired Sexual and Bladder Function

This complication may arise after open and laparoscopic rectal resection. Sympathetic and parasympathetic nerve injury may result in sexual and urinary dysfunction. Sexual dysfunction can develop in 30–50% of patients. Males with sexual dysfunction from nerve injury may develop impotence or retrograde ejaculation. Women experience loss of vaginal lubrication, and inability to achieve orgasm. Increased age and tumor penetration are risk factors for sexual dysfunction. Neurogenic bladder resulting from nerve injury is much less prevalent (5 10%). The introduction of the TME technique, as well as increased efforts to preserve the autonomic pelvic nerves during surgery, has lowered the incidence of these complications.

Data comparing sexual and bladder dysfunction between open and laparoscopic approaches are very limited. Bladder dysfunction rate is most likely the same; however, a nonsignificant trend toward increased male sexual dysfunction after laparoscopic rectal resection was recently reported. This finding warrants additional studies.

Post Anterior Resection Syndrome

Post anterior resection syndrome refers to a disorder of abnormal evacuation occurring in patients that have undergone an anterior resection of the colon. Symptoms include frequent bowel movements, incontinence of flatus and feces, urgency, and incomplete evacuation. These symptoms are attributed to the replacement of the native rectal reservoir into a more proximal portion of the colon, decreased rectal volume, and changes in rectal wall compliance induced by radiation (see Chap. 3, Radiation Proctopathy). These symptoms may gradually improve over time and are less prominent when a colonic reservoir is created (colonic pouch, coloplasty, or a Baker anastomosis). In some patients, symptoms of post anterior resection syndrome may result in severe debility.

Warning Signs for Complications

The most dreaded complication of laparoscopic anterior colorectal resection is an anastomotic leak. Signs of anastomotic leakage generally occur several days after the surgery. These include fever, abdominal distension, and the appearance of a cloudy fluid in the abdominal drains. Treatment for anastomotic leakage consists of fluid replacement, bowel rest, and antibiotics. In some cases, operative intervention with stoma construction is required.

Clinical Pearls

Improved short-term outcomes have been demonstrated in several studies of laparoscopic rectal resection. However, these procedures lengthen the time spent in the operating room in performance of the surgery. In addition, data on laparoscopic resection for low and mid rectal cancer are still limited and based mainly on retrospective studies.

It is advised that laparoscopic rectal resection for rectal cancer should be performed by highly experienced surgeons. The benefit vs. disadvantages of this technique will be further elucidated in future clinical trials.

Chapter 21
Surgery for Rectal Cancer

Shmuel Avital

Introduction

The rectum is approximately 18 cm in length and is divided into the upper intraperitoneal third and the lower extraperitoneal two-thirds. The surgical approach and clinical outcome of upper rectal tumors are similar to cancer of the colon.

As opposed to colon and upper rectal cancer, surgery for locally advanced low and mid rectal cancer has been associated with high local recurrence rates, reportedly as high as 30% until the late 1990s. Two factors that have contributed to a substantial decrease in the local recurrence rate following surgery for locally advanced rectal cancer are completion therapy with radiation, and the adoption of a surgical technique, total mesorectal excision (TME), pioneered by Dr. Bill Heald. Radiation used to be administered after the operation (termed adjuvant radiotherapy) but is now generally given prior to surgery (called neoadjuvant radiotherapy).

Evaluation prior to surgery should include full colonoscopy to rule out synchronous polyps or tumors, CT scan of the chest and abdomen, and/or positive emission tomography (PET scanning) to rule out distant metastasis. Local tumor invasion is evaluated either by transrectal ultrasound (TRUS) or by MRI. Patients with Locally advanced tumors (tumor invades beyond the muscular layer [T3 tumors] or positive local lymph nodes [N positive]) are referred to neoadjuvant treatments, as previously described.

S. Avital, MD (✉)
Chief of Surgery, Department of Surgery B, Meir Medical Center, Kfar-Saba, Israel
e-mail: avitalshmuel@gmail.com

E.D. Ehrenpreis et al. (eds.), *Anal and Rectal Diseases: A Concise Manual*,
DOI 10.1007/978-1-4614-1102-4_21, © Springer Science+Business Media, LLC 2012

General Description

There are several surgical approaches used for rectal cancer. The choice of a surgical procedure depends on the distance of the lower margin of the tumor from the anal verge and the tumor's depth of invasion. Three main options are available.

Anterior Resection

Anterior resection refers to resection of the rectum and reconstruction with anastomosis of the proximal colon to the distal rectal stump or anal canal. The procedure involves ligation of the inferior mesenteric artery (IMA) in its origin (high ligation) or ligation of the IMA after division of the left colic artery or sigmoid arteries (low ligation) and proximal transaction of the colon at the level of the distal left colon. Distal dissection is performed according to the principles of TME, meaning dissecting in planes that enable complete removal of the mesorectum. Distal transection should be at least 1 cm distal to the tumor. Reconstruction is usually performed by a circular stapler.

Abdominoperineal Resection (APR)

With APR, the entire rectum as well as the anal canal is resected. This procedure is reserved for very distal rectal tumors when adequate distal margins cannot be achieved without damaging the anal sphincters and in patients who already have sphincter malfunctions.

The principles of APR are the same as for anterior resection. The rectum is dissected to the pelvic floor but is not transected distally. Thereafter, the anal canal is dissected from the perineal skin, up and beyond the pelvic floor, to where the rectum is removed en bloc with the anus. The proximal end of the colon is exteriorized as a permanent end stoma in the left lower abdomen. The perineum is sutured closed.

Local Excision

Local excision is reserved for low rectal tumors in cases of early tumors with a favorable histology (tumors less than 3 cm in diameter, no submucosal invasion (T1), well differentiated, and no lymphatic or vascular invasion). Other indications include more invasive tumors in patients with severe comorbidities who are not able to undergo major surgery. The operation is performed via the anal canal with specific retractors. Adequate circumferential and deep margins are essential. The cavity created may be closed with absorbable sutures. For high lesions (beyond 8 cm from the anal verge), when transanal excision is not possible or is too difficult, transanal endoscopic microsurgery (TEM) may be used. TEM consists of a long rectoscope connected to a fiberoptic system, which uses CO_2 insufflation and long surgical instruments. This system allows adequate resection of high rectal lesions.

Goals of Surgery

The goals of surgery are to achieve negative histological distal margins with complete removal of the rectum with its mesenteric roots (i.e., IMA) and its mesorectum.

It is important to dissect the mesorectum along its embroyenal planes ("the holey plane") as an accurate dissection is associated with low local recurrence.

Indications

The primary indication for surgery is rectal cancer with local or regional disease. Patients with distant metastatic disease should be evaluated for metastasis resectability.

Patients with metastases, which are potentially resectable (limited liver metastasis), should be considered for a combination of chemotherapy and surgery. Surgery is usually performed in two stages (the rectum first and then the metastatic disease).

Palliative surgery for pain, bleeding, tenesmus, and incontinence may improve quality of life in patients with metastatic disease.

Contraindications

Patients with severe comorbidities who are unfit to undergo major surgery.

Relative Contraindications

Less severe comorbidities requiring judgment regarding risks and benefits from the surgeon and patient.

Alternatives

As a general rule, surgical resection is the key to potential cure in rectal cancer. However, following neoadjuvant radiotherapy, pathological reports demonstrate as high as a 15% complete elimination of tumor in resected specimens. Complete clinical response following radiotherapyis a good prognostic sign, however, it is recommended that these patients should also undergo surgery. Radiochemotherapy alone or in combination with local excision should be considered in patients who are unfit to undergo major surgery.

Outcomes

Generally, local recurrence and survival are related to pathological stage of the disease. For all patients, disease-free 5-year survival averages 60–70%. Overall survival is approximately 75%. Stage I patients have close to 100% disease-free survival, Stage II between 70 and 80%, and Stage III between 50 and 60% disease-free survival. Local recurrence, a major concern in rectal cancer, ranges from 3 to 15%. Factors associated with decreased local recurrence are increased tumor distance from the anal verge (with the lowest local recurrence for upper rectal tumors), use of a TME surgical approach, and the use of adjuvant radiotherapy. Neoadjuvant radiotherapy results in decreased local recurrence when compared to patients undergoing adjuvant radiotherapy.

Important Complications

Intraoperative Bleeding

Major bleeding can arise from the presacral venous complex. This might be very difficult to control. Surgical management consists of thumbtacks, occluder pins, clips, and packing.

Anastomotic Leak

Leak rates vary from 2 to 10%. Clinical manifestations of leaks may vary from local infection to fulminant sepsis. Low anastomoses and neoadjuvant radiotherapy are associated with an increased leak rate. In these cases, it is recommended to construct a diverting ileostomy initially. This substantially lowers the consequences of postoperative leaks and is typically reversed 6–12 weeks after surgery.

Wound Infections

These may develop in 10–20% of patients and are usually managed with drainage and antibiotics. Unhealed perineal wounds following APR may occur in up to 25% of patients. In some cases, management may include surgical intervention.

Sexual and Urinary Dysfunction

Sympathetic and parasympathetic nerve injury may cause sexual and urinary dysfunction. Sexual dysfunction can develop in 30–50% of patients. In males, sexual dysfunction manifests as impotence or retrograde ejaculation. In females, it presents as loss of lubrication or inability to achieve orgasm. Increased age and degree of tumor penetration into nerves are risk factors. Nerve injury causing neurogenic bladder is much less prevalent (5–10%). Introduction of the TME technique and efforts to preserve the autonomic pelvic nerves during surgery have helped to lower the incidence of these complications.

Post Anterior Resection Syndrome

Post anterior resection syndrome refers to symptoms related to evacuation. These symptoms include urgency, frequent bowel movements, fecal incontinence, perineal pain and discomfort, and tenesmus. These symptoms are attributed to decreased rectal capacity and to radiation-induced reduction of rectal compliance. These symptoms generally gradually improve with time and are less prominent when a colonic reservoir is created in during surgery (colonic pouch, coloplasty, or a Baker anastomosis).

Clinical Pearls

The optimal treatment for curable rectal cancer is usually a combination of preoperative radiotherapy followed by surgery. The TME technique, with preservation of the autonomic pelvic nerves, is associated with low local recurrence and fewer postoperative complications. In early tumors, local excision may be an optional surgical approach.

Lower stage and upper rectal tumors are associated with better prognosis.

Chapter 22
Surgical Colostomy and Ileostomy

Marc Singer and Shmuel Avital

Description of Procedures

An enterostomy, or stoma, may be constructed from either the ileum (ileostomy) or the colon (colostomy). Fashioning a stoma involves bringing the intestine through the anterior abdominal wall. This allows intestinal contents to drain through the stoma and into an appliance. A variety of appliances are now available to suit the particular needs of each patient and their specific stoma. The two broad categories of stoma construction are "end" stomas and "loop" or "diverting" stomas. Stomas may also be temporary or permanent, depending on the indication for stoma construction and medical status of the patient.

Indications

Stomas are indicated if there is a need to divert the flow of enteric contents. There are a variety of reasons for stoma requirement. Some cancer operations, such as abdominoperineal resection, require the permanent removal of the anorectum, thus necessitating a permanent colostomy. Other operations, such as a low anterior resection, (with a colorectal or coloanal anastomosis), often require a temporary diverting stoma. Most commonly, a loop ileostomy is utilized in this setting. Temporarily

M. Singer, MD (✉)
Department of Surgery, Division of Colon and Rectal Surgery, NorthShore University Health System, 2650 Ridge Avenue, Ste 2507, Evanston, IL 60201, USA
e-mail: msinger1@northshore.org

S. Avital, MD
Chief of Surgery, Department of Surgery B, Meir Medical Center, Kfar-Saba, Israel

E.D. Ehrenpreis et al. (eds.), *Anal and Rectal Diseases: A Concise Manual*,
DOI 10.1007/978-1-4614-1102-4_22, © Springer Science+Business Media, LLC 2012

diverting the fecal stream is required while healing of an anastomosis takes place. This is an important consideration in the setting of preoperative radiation therapy or anastomosis distal to the midrectum. Penetrating abdominal trauma, such as stab or gunshot wounds, may require temporary stoma placement while damaged gastrointestinal organs are healing. Patients with intestinal conditions such as Crohn's disease may require temporary stomas during medical management of severe flares. However, these patients may ultimately require permanent stomas depending on the outcome of medical and surgical treatment of the primary disease. Patients with fecal incontinence or severe constipation may require stoma placement as primary therapy. Complex pelvic operations, such repair of a rectovaginal fistula, occasionally also require proximal diversion. Diversion of the fecal stream to assist with healing of a sacral decubitus ulcer may be required. Patients with neurological disorders or paralyzed patients may benefit from a stoma for severe constipation or fecal incontinence. Emergency stomas may also be required for patients with toxic megacolon or severe pseudomembranous colitis. When resection and anastomosis are not a safe surgical choice (such as in the setting of perforated diverticulitis or other perforations in an unprepared colon), a stoma may be required. Construction of an anastomosis is also avoided in patients with peritonitis, hemodynamic instability, and severe malnutrition, due to high rates of anastomotic failure.

Contraindications

Contraindications include medical morbidities precluding anesthesia (however, stoma construction may be performed under regional anesthesia). Under limited circumstances, a diverting loop transverse colostomy can even be performed under local anesthesia in unstable patients. Relative contraindications to stoma construction include the inability of the patient to perform postoperative stoma care, and/or lack of access to care and appliances. The presence of neurologic disabilities or limited use of the hands (such as in patients with severe rheumatoid arthritis) may preclude the ability to care for the stoma or change appliances. Such patients will require nursing care and, in some circumstances, inpatient treatment at a nursing or long-term care facility. These problems do not preclude stoma placement if otherwise indicated, but such issues should be considered and addressed prior to the operation to the greatest extent possible.

Alternatives

The alternatives to a stoma depend on the specific indication and disease state of a particular patient. For example, patients with fecal incontinence often can be successfully managed with a medical regimen, and at times, sphincter reconstruction.

Patients with ulcerative colitis often elect to undergo a proctocolectomy and ileoanal anastomosis rather than permanent ileostomy. Patients with cancer can choose to undergo alternative treatments, but typically the cancer operation dictates the further care and need for stoma placement. Patients with Crohn's disease may delay surgical resection and pursue medical therapy.

How the Operation Is Performed

Stomas may be constructed in a variety of ways. One of the most critical factors for creating a well-functioning stoma occurs before the patient comes to the operating room. In the elective setting, preoperative consultation with an enterostomal therapist is critical. The therapist will review the type of stoma planned. He or she will then examine the patient in the supine, standing, and sitting positions. The position of the patient's pants, abdominal folds, abdominal scars, etc., will be noted. As a general rule, a stoma should be located at the apex of the infraumbilical fold, at the level of the rectus muscle. This is the starting point for identifying an ideal location for a stoma and must be modified for each patient. The appliance requires a flat surface so that an adequate seal can be formed with the skin. This means that the stoma should not be located at a fold or crease. The site should not be too close to the umbilicus. If possible, the stoma should not be near an open wound. It should also not be positioned at the same level where a patient wears his or her pants/belt. The stoma therapist will also provide education to the patient, and their family or caretakers. This education session typically includes demonstrations with photos and other tools related to the use of an appliance. Although time consuming, these sessions afford the patient and their providers an opportunity to fully understand postoperative stoma care. Preoperative evaluation by a stoma therapist may not be possible when the procedure is performed in an emergency situation such as colonic trauma or perforation.

Stoma construction may be performed in an open or laparoscopic fashion. The critical elements are essentially the same. An ileostomy should be constructed distally, so as to allow maximal absorption. However, the ileostomy should not be so close to the ileocecal valve that will make closure complicated, since adequate mobilization for this portion of the colon may be difficult. Typically, the ileostomy is constructed 10–20 cm proximal to the ileocecal valve. The site of the colostomy depends on the indication for the procedure, but most the common colostomies are from the sigmoid or descending colon or are loop transverse colostomies.

The stoma site on the abdominal wall is prepared by excising a circular disk of skin and subcutaneous fat. This should be matched to the size of the bowel. The fascia should be incised in a cruciate fashion. The rectus fibers are separated, but not divided, and the posterior sheath is also incised in a cruciate fashion. It is difficult to know the exact size of the orifice, but as a general rule, two fingers should be able to comfortably pass through the orifice.

An end stoma involves division of the bowel, followed by passage of the cut end of the proximal bowel through the abdominal wall. The distal end may possibly be left free in the abdomen. Maturation of the stoma depends on the stomal effluent. Descending sigmoid colostomies have relatively solid output, therefore should be matured so they are flush with the skin. The solid effluent is unlikely to be toxic to the skin at the colostomy site. Therefore, the colostomy can be constructed in this manner. The diverted ileum should be matured in an everted, or "Brooke," fashion. The end of the bowel is carried through the abdominal wall, and then everted onto itself. It is then secured to the dermis. Eversion of the ileum at the ostomy site prevents the development of serositis (a potential cause of high ostomy output) and also allows for proper sealing of the appliance. The ileostomy effluent is highly caustic to the skin. Significant skin inflammation and excoriation can occur in less than 24 h after stoma placement if there is exposed skin between the stoma and the appliance wafer. The everted stoma allows for direct apposition of the wafer to the stoma and therefore completely conceals and protects adjacent skin from damage.

If it is necessary to vent the distal bowel (e.g., in distal obstructions, or when there is excessive colonic mucous production), the distal portion of the bowel may be brought through a separate wound as a mucus fistula or thorough the same wound as the end stoma. This is known as a divided loop stoma, end loop, or a "double barrel" stoma. It functions as a loop stoma, but constructed as an end stoma, and therefore meets the definition of an "end loop."

A loop stoma is constructed by bringing a segment of bowel through the abdominal wound. The bowel is divided outside the abdomen and then matured. The functional limb should occupy the large majority of the opening, while the nonfunctional (distal) limb should take up only a small portion of the wound. This serves to vent the distal bowel and also secures the bowel to the wound. This means that at subsequent closure, a local operation at the site of the stoma can be performed, making a laparotomy unnecessary. If the distal limb is left in the abdomen, a full laparotomy is required to perform the anastomoses.

As described above, an end loop stoma is constructed as a loop; however, the distal limb is a short blind pouch. It is an end stoma functionally, but called an end loop because it is constructed as a loop.

Regardless of the type of stoma produced, absorbable sutures should be used in constructing the stoma. The appliance should be applied immediately on completion of the surgery. The stoma should not be matured until any other abdominal wounds are closed, to minimize contamination and reduce the chance of developing a wound infection at the stoma site.

Outcomes

Outcomes of stoma placement is dependent on the indication for stoma (cancer, IBD, trauma).

Complications

Early complications include bleeding and infection at the stoma site. Local infection can result in a mucocutaneous separation at the edge of the stoma. This can usually be treated with local wound care with subsequent healing. Retractions of the stoma may occur if there is tension on the bowel. Ischemia may occur as a result. It is not uncommon the stoma to appear congested, or ischemic after surgery. An endoscope or even a transparent test tube may be inserting into the stoma to visualize the bowel at the level of the fascia.

Later complications included prolapse of the stoma and parastomal hernia. The incidence of these depends on the type of stoma produced. The chance of eventual development of a parastomal hernia is high (upwards of 50%). In fact, surgical texts suggest that all stomas will eventually develop herniation if patients live long enough. Recently, there have been reports on mesh implantation at the time of the initial stoma formation in cases of permanent stoma placement to prevent the development of parastomal hernias. Despite the theoretical risk of mesh infection, these reports have demonstrated a high success rate with very few cases of mesh infection.

Local skin irritations are the most common complications of stomas. This may require changing the type of pouches, barriers, and/or skin products. Peristomal fistulization may occur in patients with IBD, while stomal varices can be seen in patients with cirrhosis of the liver.

High ostomy output may occur with when ostomy construction is combined with small intestinal resection and/or if the ostomy is placed in the proximal ileum or jejunum. Previous small intestinal resection or active small intestinal disease is associated with high ostomy output. Normally, the output in a mature ileostomy is less than 1 L daily. Consequences of high ostomy output include fluid and electrolyte disturbances, malabsorption, and weight loss. Treatment includes attention to fluids, electrolytes, and nutrition and inhibition of gastric secretions with acid blocking drugs. Treatment of underlying intestinal disease and administration of antimotility agents are also of potential benefit. Another option is administration of subcutaneous injection of the somatostatin analog octreotide, as it reduces small intestinal secretions.

Clinical Pearls

Patients with well-placed stomas can lead full and independent lives. They should be counseled that stoma patients can work, travel, enjoy sports, perform sexual activities, etc., without limitation. Many patients avoid colon cancer screening due to the fears of requiring a stoma from the findings or complications of colonoscopy. This should never be an impediment to screening or appropriate care. Close cooperation with an enterostomal therapist is critical to achieve successful results of stoma placement. Stoma complications directly affect the quality of life of patients. Proper construction and strict attention to details of placement and management will result in improved outcomes.

Chapter 23
Surgery for Rectal Foreign Bodies

Marc Singer and Shmuel Avital

Description of Procedures

The majority of retained foreign bodies can be extracted though the anus. A detailed history should be elicited. Patients are frequently uncomfortable discussing the circumstances and should be interviewed privately. Some objects may present a risk to the physician, such as broken glass (glass thermometers, light bulbs, and jars), and this should be specifically queried. Extraction may be performed in the office or emergency department, but often requires sedation and local anesthesia. Rarely, an abdominal procedure (laparotomy or laparoscopy) is required to remove foreign bodies. Spontaneous evacuation is prevented in many cases because insertion of the object causes spasm of the anal sphincter. Furthermore, the size and shape of the object may never allow for spontaneous relaxation of the sphincters to a diameter large enough to accommodate evacuation.

Indications

Most retained foreign bodies should be extracted. Small and smooth objects (marbles and rings) may be observed. If there is any concern that the foreign body is too large to pass, or may create a rectal injury, then it must be extracted. Retained objects

M. Singer, MD (✉)
Department of Surgery, Division of Colon and Rectal Surgery, NorthShore University Health System, 2650 Ridge Avenue, Ste 2507, Evanston, IL 60201, USA
e-mail: msinger1@northshore.org

S. Avital, MD
Chief of Surgery, Department of Surgery B, Meir Medical Center, Kfar-Saba, Israel

E.D. Ehrenpreis et al. (eds.), *Anal and Rectal Diseases: A Concise Manual*,
DOI 10.1007/978-1-4614-1102-4_23, © Springer Science+Business Media, LLC 2012

often cause pain, but even if asymptomatic, erosion through the rectal wall may occur, resulting in bleeding and/or perforation. If a perforation of the rectum or colon occurs, then a laparotomy or laparoscopy may be required for extraction, definitive repair, washout, or proximal diversion. Timing of the injury may determine the need for an abdominal procedure. Peritonitis or pneumoperitoneum suggests an intraperitoneal injury, raising the likelihood of an abdominal procedure.

Contraindications

Patients with contraindications to anesthesia may be unable to undergo sedation. Patients on anticoagulants should be considered for reversal with fresh frozen plasma if mucosal trauma is highly suspected (e.g., broken glass in rectum).

Alternatives

A trial of observation is appropriate in selected patients. If patients are asymptomatic, and the object is small, observation is considered appropriate. Abdominal and pelvic radiography can help to assess the size and type of the retained object(s), and predict if spontaneous evacuation will be possible. If the patient is symptomatic, or a perforation has occurred, then a laparotomy or laparoscopic exploration of the abdomen may be indicated.

How the Operation Is Performed

Abdominal and pelvic X-rays should be obtained in order to identify the nature, number, and locations of objects, and also to rule out pneumoperitnoneum. Some objects may not be visible if they are not radiopaque (plastic, organic matter such as vegetables). Transanal recovery of foreign bodies may be performed in the office/ emergency department in selected patients. A thorough digital examination should be performed first. The examiner should be cautious not to push objects proximally while inserting a finger into the rectum. The examiner should also avoid injury by sharp objects (pencils and screwdrivers) or broken glass (light bulbs). If the object is in the distal rectum, manual extraction may be accomplished. If not, then an anoscope such as a Hill-Ferguson or a bivalve anoscope is carefully inserted into the anus. The rectum is then inspected. If the object can be visualized, then it should be retrieved with a clamp. However, when visualization cannot be achieved, or the object is too large to pass through the sphincters (which often may be in spasm), bringing the patient to the operating room is advised.

There are several benefits of performing the extraction of foreign bodies in the operating room. Patients can receive conscious sedation or placed under general anesthesia.

This will improve patient comfort and will also allow for thorough relaxation of the sphincters. The full array of anoscopes, proctoscopes, flexible endoscopes, and grasping instruments should be available in the operating room to facilitate extraction. Finally, if a rectal injury, especially bleeding, was to occur during extraction, the operating room is the ideal place for the control of such injuries.

Conscious sedation, regional anesthesia, or general anesthesia is utilized according to the preference of patient and surgeon. Positioning the patient in prone jackknife position will allow for greatest exposure of the anorectum; however, many surgeons prefer the lithotomy positioning. This allows the surgeon to apply abdominal pressure to facilitate extraction, or conversion to a laparotomy/laparoscopic exploration of the abdomen if needed. Injection of local anesthetic into the sphincter itself should be performed regardless of the type of sedation used. This will allow for maximal sphincter dilation. The sphincter can be safely dilated to 40 mm diameter or more in most patients with appropriate sedation and local anesthesia.

Formal anoscopy and/or rigid proctoscopy are then performed. If the object is visualized, it should be grasped with a ring forceps or proctoscopic biopsy forceps if possible. If the object occupies the entire lumen of the rectum, then a suction effect is created as downward traction is applied. In such cases, a Foley catheter may be carefully guided proximally, past the object, and air insufflated into the proximal colon. This will break the suction and will gently push the object distally by creating positive pressure. This technique is also helpful for objects that cannot easily be grasped with clamps such as jars and bottles.

Flexible endoscopy can be helpful in retrieving objects that have migrated proximally into the sigmoid or descending colon. Minimal air should be insufflated to avoid pushing the object more proximally. A jumbo biopsy forceps or wire snare can be used to retrieve the objects.

Once retrieved, objects should be inspected for sharp edges, missing parts, etc. Proctoscopy (rigid or flexible) should be repeated to evaluate the bowel for injuries. Postoperative radiography must be obtained to assess for the presence of pneumoperitoneum. If there is any concern based on the clinical examination X-ray, a CT scan or a contrast enema should be immediately performed to definitively exclude a perforation.

If an object cannot be retrieved by these described techniques, a laparotomy or laparoscopic exploration should be performed. It may be possible to manipulate the object from within the abdomen toward the anus. If this is not successful, then a colostomy must be performed. This should be the maneuver of last choice as it puts the patient at risk of abscess and fistula formation.

Outcomes

Generally, objects will be successfully retrieved by one of the methods described previously. There are rarely any long-term sequelae of rectal foreign bodies. Sphincter injury due to insertion trauma will be discussed in a separate chapter.

Complications

Complications may occur during insertion of objects. These complications include local irritation, fissures, or even anal sphincter injuries. The extent of insertion injuries depends on the size of the object and the degree of force of insertion. Injury to the rectum may cause bleeding. Full-thickness perforation may occur during insertion, during removal, or secondary to mucosal erosion if there is a delay until extraction takes place. If perforation occurs, and there is significant postponement, some patients may require a colostomy. An extraperitoneal perforation can usually be treated with drainage and antibiotics.

Warning Signs for Complications

Patients may experience ongoing bleeding, pain, fever, vomiting, or diarrhea if an abscess or peritonitis is present. Fecal incontinence may be possible if the sphincter was injured at the time of foreign body insertion or extraction.

Clinical Pearls

A thorough history should be obtained in confidence. Patients should be specifically questioned about what object(s) have been inserted. This will gauge the degree of clinical suspicion for rectal injury. In addition, it is important to consider the possibility that multiple objects are present. Any suspicion that retained foreign bodies are a result of rape or physical abuse should prompt immediate referral to law enforcement professions and social services.

Chapter 24
Anesthesia for Anorectal Surgery

Shmuel Avital

Introduction

Anorectal surgery requires deep anesthesia since this region of the body has a dense sensory nerve supply and is highly reflexogenic. Surgical procedures under light anesthesia will result in intense pain, reflexive body movements, tachypnea, and even laryngeal spasm.

Deep anesthesia for anorectal procedures can be achieved using different forms of anesthesia including general endotracheal, regional, or local anesthesia; local anesthesia is generally administered in conjunction with general sedation.

Many anorectal procedures can be safely and cost-effectively performed using local anesthesia. The use of local anesthetic methods is safer with relatively fewer complications compared to other anesthetic techniques. However, regional and general anesthesia can be used depending upon patient or physician preference.

A variety of factors should be considered when selecting the choice of anesthesia for anorectal procedures. For major operations such as rectal resection, general anesthesia is preferred, since deep general anesthesia enables abdominal muscle relaxation with no response to surgical stimuli. Concerns regarding airway management may preclude the use of conscious sedation for procedures performed in the prone position. A combination of light and general anesthesia with some form of regional blockade can be extended into the postoperative period for management of postoperative pain.

S. Avital, MD (✉)
Chief of Surgery, Department of Surgery B, Meir Medical Center, Kfar-Saba, Israel
e-mail: avitalshmuel@gmail.com

E.D. Ehrenpreis et al. (eds.), *Anal and Rectal Diseases: A Concise Manual*,
DOI 10.1007/978-1-4614-1102-4_24, © Springer Science+Business Media, LLC 2012

Local Anesthesia

Local anesthetic mixtures typically involve combinations of lidocaine, bupivacaine, and epinephrine. Local anesthesia may be performed by posterior perineal block or by the use local injections. Using the posterior perineal block, anesthesia is achieved by two levels of injections based on the direction of anal canal innervation. Initially, an injection of local anesthetic is directed into the presacral area to anesthetize the superficial posterior nerve branches. This is then followed by deeper and lateral injections to anesthetize the pudendal nerves.

Local nonanatomical anesthesia has also been described. Injection typically starts in the perianal skin and then progresses deeper toward the anorectal ring. Since the anoderm is an extremely sensitive area, sedation of the patient should precede initial perianal skin injections. Perianal infiltration of local anesthesia is a relatively simple procedure and can achieve full relaxation of the anal canal. Injection of local anesthesia can be accomplished in under 5 min, and the procedure can begin almost immediately thereafter.

Another technique associated with less pain production has been reported. This technique involves injection of the anesthetic solution a few millimeters proximal to the dentate line, into a significantly less sensitive area, followed by squeezing the injected solution toward the distal anal canal. Subsequent injections are then administered distally into the newly anesthetized areas. This technique essentially reverses of the steps usually taken with conventional injection techniques.

Despite concerns regarding the use of sedation and local anesthesia in patients operated in the prone position, there are some reports demonstrating its feasibility. Patients may be placed in the prone position and then receive intravenous narcotics. Subsequent injection of a short-acting local anesthetic causes stimulation that, to some extent, may counteract respiratory depression caused by the intravenous anesthetic. The operation may then proceed with careful monitoring by the anesthesiologist. Close coordination between the surgeon and the anesthesiologist or anesthetist is of paramount importance when using this method.

Spinal Anesthesia

This technique is relatively simple, rapidly effective, and may achieve deep local anesthesia with good postoperative pain relief. However, spinal anesthesia is associated with intraoperative side effects including hypotension and bradycardia. Postoperative side effects consist of postdural puncture headache and transitory radicular irritation.

Caudal Anesthesia

With caudal anesthesia, a local anesthetic is injected into the caudal canal through the sacral hiatus. The caudal canal lies distal to the dura of the spinal cord that terminates at the level of S2 and consists of areolar connective tissue, fat, sacral nerves, lymphatics, and a rich venous plexus. Caudal anesthesia produces blockage of the sacral and lumbar nerve roots. A combination of light general anesthesia with caudal block may achieve a high level of postoperative pain relief. Other advantages include a readily predictable level of anesthesia, decreased sensory and motor block in the legs, and fewer systemic complications (such as drop in blood pressure, or postdural puncture headache) compared to spinal anesthesia. However, in some adults, anatomic considerations preclude the use of this procedure.

General Anesthesia

A significant advantage of general anesthesia is its rapid induction. Additionally, general anesthesia provides high quality sedation, amnesia, analgesia, and muscle relaxation, with limited intraoperative cardiorespiratory side effects. However, postoperative nausea and vomiting are relatively common. In addition, the analgesic effects of general anesthesia are limited to the early postoperative period such that overall patient recovery time may be prolonged compared to other methods of anesthesia due to the necessity for introduction of additional medications for pain control.

Suggested Reading

Textbooks

Barnes L, Corman ML, editors. Colon and Rectal Surgery. 4th ed. Philadelphia, PA: Lippincott–Raven Publishers, 1998.

Fazio VW, Church JM, Delaney CP. Current therapy in colon and rectal surgery. 2nd edition. Elsevier Mosby. 2005. 212–217.

Feldman M, Friedman LS, Sleisenger MH, editors. Sleisenger & Fordtran's Gastrointestinal and Liver Disease. 7th ed. Philadelphia, PA: Saunders, 2002.

Gordon PH, Nivatvongs S, editors. Principles and Practice of Surgery for the Colon, Rectum and Anus. 2nd ed. New York, NY: Marcel Dekker, 1999.

Gorbach SL, Bartlett JG, Blacklow NR, editors. Infectious Diseases. 2nd ed. Philadelphia, PA: Saunders, 1997.

Yamada T, editor. Textbook of Gastroenterology. 2nd ed. Philadelphia, PA: Lippincott Williams & Wilkins, 1995.

Review Articles

Bartram C. Dynamic evaluation of the anorectum. Radiol Clin North Am 2003;41(2):425–41.

Bharucha AE. Fecal incontinence. Gastroenterology 2003;124(6):1672–85.

Gopal DV. Diseases of the rectum and anus: a clinical approach to common disorders. Clin Cornerstone 2002;4(4):34–48.

Hong JJ, Park W, Ehrenpreis ED. Review article: current therapeutic options for radiation proctopathy. Aliment Pharmacol Ther 2001;15(9):1253–62.

Maria G, Sganga G, Civello IM, Brisinda G. Botulinum neurotoxin and other treatments for fissure-in-ano and pelvic floor disorders. B J Surg 2002;89(8):950–61.

Moore HG, Guillem JG. Anal neoplasms. Surg Clin North Am. 2002;82(6):1233–51.

Moore HG, Guillem JG. Multimodality management of locally advanced rectal cancer. Am Surg 2003;69(7):612–9.

McLaughlin SD, Clark SK, Tekkis PP, Ciclitira PJ, Nicholls RJ. Review article: restorative proctocolectomy, indications, management of complications and follow-up – a guide for gastroenterologists. Aliment Pharmacol Ther 2008;27, 895–909.

Madiba TE, Baig MK, Wexner SD. Surgical management of rectal prolapse. Arch Surg 2005;140: 63–73.

E.D. Ehrenpreis et al. (eds.), *Anal and Rectal Diseases: A Concise Manual*,
DOI 10.1007/978-1-4614-1102-4, © Springer Science+Business Media, LLC 2012

Nelson R. Anorectal abscess fistula: what do we know? Surg Clin North Am 2002;82(6):1139–51.

Olsen AL, Rao SS. Clinical neurophysiology and electrodiagnostic testing of the pelvic floor. Gastroenterol Clin North Am 2001;30(1):33–54,v–vi.

Schmitt SL, Wexner SD. Treatment of anorectal manifestations of AIDS. Int J STD AIDS 1994;5(1):8–10.

Utzig MJ, Kroesen AJ, Buhr HJ. Concepts in pathogenesis and treatment of chronic anal fissure – a review of the literature. Am J Gastroenterol 2003;98(5):968–74.

Wald A. Anorectal and pelvic pain in women: diagnostic considerations and treatment. J Clin Gastroenterol 2001;33(4):283–8.

Journal Articles

Barisic GI, Krivokapic ZV, Markovic VA, Popovic MA. Outcome of overlapping anal sphincter repair after 3 months and after a mean of 80 months. Int J Colorectal Dis 2006;21(1):52–6

Efron JE, Corman ML, Fleshman J, Barnett J, Nagle D, Birnbaum E, Weiss EG, Nogueras JJ, Sligh S, Rabine J, Wexner SD. Safety and effectiveness of temperature-controlled radio-frequency energy delivery to the anal canal (Secca procedure) for the treatment of fecal incontinence. Dis Colon Rectum 2003;46(12):1606–16; discussion 1616–8.

Elsebae MM. A study of fecal incontinence in patients with chronic anal fissure: prospective, randomized, controlled trial of the extent of internal anal sphincter division during lateral sphincterotomy. World J Surg 2007;31(10):2052–7.

Felt-Bersma RJF, Stella MTE, Cuesta MA. Rectal prolapse, rectal intussusception, rectocele, solitary rectal ulcer syndrome, and enterocele. Gastroenterol Clin N Am 2008;37:645–668.

Nivatvongs S. Technique of local anesthesia for anorectal surgery. Dis Colon Rectum 1997;40(9):1128–9.

Grey BR, Sheldon RR, Telford KJ, Kiff ES. Anterior anal sphincter repair can be of long term benefit: a 12-year case cohort from a single surgeon. BMC Surg 2007;11;7:1.

Gudaityte J, Marchertiene I, Pavalkis D. Anesthesia for ambulatory anorectal surgery. Medicina (Kaunas) 2004;40(2):101–11.

Hancke E, Rikas E, Suchan K, Völke K. Dermal flap coverage for chronic anal fissure: lower incidence of anal incontinence compared to lateral internal sphincterotomy after long-term follow-up. Dis Colon Rectum 2010;53(11):1563–8.

Hetzer FH, Hahnloser D, Clavien PA, Demartines N. Quality of life and morbidity after permanent sacral nerve stimulation for fecal incontinence. Arch Surg 2007;142(1):8–13.

McGuire BB, Brannigan AE, O'Connell PR. Ileal pouch–anal anastomosis. Br J Surg 2007;94:812–823.

Joshi GP, Neugebauer EA; PROSPECT Collaboration. Evidence-based management of pain after haemorrhoidectomy surgery. Br J Surg 2010;97(8):1155–68.

Li S, Coloma M, White PF, Watcha MF, Chiu JW, Li H, Huber PJ Jr. Comparison of the costs and recovery profiles of three anesthetic techniques for ambulatory anorectal surgery. Anesthesiology 2000;93(5):1225–30.

McFarland EG, Fletcher JG, Pickhardt P, Dachman A, Yee J, McCollough CH, Macari M, Knechtges P, Zalis M, Barish M, Kim DH, Keysor KJ, Johnson CD; American College of Radiology. ACR Colon Cancer Committee white paper: status of CT colonography 2009. J Am Coll Radiol 2009;6(11):756–772.e4.

Malouf AJ, Vaizey CJ, Nicholls RJ, Kamm MA. Permanent sacral nerve stimulation for fecal incontinence. Ann Surg 2000;232(1):143–8.

Matsuoka H, Mavrantonis C, Wexner SD, Oliveira L, Gilliland R, Pikarsky A. Postanal repair for fecal incontinence--is it worthwhile? Dis Colon Rectum 2000;43(11):1561–7.

Menteş BB, Tezcaner T, Yilmaz U, Leventoğlu S, Oguz M. Results of lateral internal sphinctero-tomy for chronic anal fissure with particular reference to quality of life. Dis Colon Rectum 2006;49(7):1045–51.

Nyam DC, Pemberton JH. Long-term results of lateral internal sphincterotomy for chronic anal fissure with particular reference to incidence of fecal incontinence. Dis Colon Rectum 1999;42(10):1306–10.

Read TE, Henry SE, Hovis RM, Fleshman JW, Birnbaum EH, Caushaj PF, Kodner IJ. Prospective evaluation of anesthetic technique for anorectal surgery. Dis Colon Rectum 2002;45(11):1553–8.

Wexner SD, Jin HY, Weiss EG, Nogueras JJ, Li VK. Factors associated with failure of the artificial bowel sphincter: a study of over 50 cases from Cleveland Clinic Florida. Dis Colon Rectum 2009;52(9):1550–7.

Zbar AP, Lienemann A, Fritsch H, Beer-Gabel M, Pescatori M. Rectocele: pathogenesis and surgi-cal management. Int J Colorectal Dis 2003;18:369–384.

Ruiz D, Pinto RA, Hull TL, Efron JE, Wexner SD. Does the Radiofrequency Procedure for Fecal Incontinence Improve Quality of Life and Incontinence at 1-Year Follow-Up? Dis Colon Rectum, July 2010; 53: 1041–1046

Index